The Economics *of* Health Reconsidered

The Economics *of* Health Reconsidered

Thomas Rice

Health Administration Press
Chicago, Illinois 1998

02   01   00   99   98   5   4   3   2

Library of Congress Cataloging-in-Publication Data
Rice, Thomas H.
   The economics of health reconsidered / by Thomas Rice.
      p.   cm.
   Includes bibliographical references and index.
   ISBN 1-56793-073-5 (alk. paper)
   1. Medical economics—Mathematical models.   2. Medical care—Cost effectiveness.   3. Medical economics—United States—Mathematical models.   I. Title.
   RA410.R53   1998
   338.4'33621—dc21   97-43076
                                                                 CIP
The paper used in this publication meets the minimum requirements of American National Standard for Information Sciences—Permanence of Paper for Printed Library Materials, ANSI Z39.48–1984.   ∞ ™

Health Administration Press
A division of the Foundation
   of the American College of
   Healthcare Executives
One North Franklin Street
Chicago, IL 60606-3491
312/424-2800

To Clara, Danny, and Kate

CONTENTS

FIGURES

TABLES

FOREWORD

SUPPOSE a family residing on the East Coast of the United States decides to visit the West Coast. The family has whittled down potential destinations to two cities: San Diego at the southern end of the state of California and Seattle at the northern end of the state of Washington. Family members who know about such things are charged with discovering, for each destination, the route that will "get the family there the fastest," that being the explicit objective posed for the navigators.

Because the navigators have been expressly given a narrow goal—to find the route that will "get the family there as quickly as possible"—we can safely call the route that does so "efficient," but only, of course, relative to that specific, narrow goal. Had the navigators been given the task of finding the route that can get the family to the destination as quickly as possible, but that also takes in at least three tourist attractions, the "most efficient" route might be somewhat different. Evidently, in abstraction from a clearly specified objective, the term "efficiency" would have little meaning in this context.

By similar logic, the most efficient route *relative to the goal of getting to Seattle in the least amount of time* would be highly inefficient if the family ultimately had agreed to sojourn to San Diego. Indeed, of the three routes, (1) the route getting the family to San Diego in the least amount of time, (2) a route that gets the family to San Diego, but not as quickly as the first route, and (3) the route that would get the family most quickly to Seattle, the last surely would be the least efficient and the worst route, if as quickly as possible to San Diego the family desired to travel.

This little lesson in road travel may strike the reader as obvious, even condescending. It may be so for readers not routinely engaged in the debate over American health policy. Alas, we cannot be sure that all of the participants in that debate would grasp this lesson or, if they did, whether they could see its relevance to human activities other than road travel. Even some highly distinguished economists who ought to know better—and at some time in their career surely did know better—can be quite cavalier in the use of the word "efficiency" in their normative pronouncements on health policy. Consider, for example, the use of that word by Milton Friedman, the widely celebrated Nobel Laureate in economics, as he ventures onto the turf of health economics and policy. In an editorial entitled "Gammon's Law Points to Health-Care Solution" that was published by the prestigious *The Wall Street Journal* (November 12, 1991), Professor Friedman, formerly of the University of Chicago and now at the Hoover Institute of Stanford University, sharply attacked the government-run Medicare program for the elderly and the Medicaid program for the disabled and the poor. He concluded thus:

> The *inefficiency,* high cost and inequitable character of our medical system can be fundamentally remedied in only one way: by moving in the other direction, toward re-privatizing medical care. . . . The [proposed] reform has two major steps: (1) End both Medicare and Medicaid and replace them with a requirement that every U.S. family unit have a major medical insurance policy with a high deductible, say $20,000 a year or 30% of the unit's income during the prior two years, whichever is lower. (2) End the tax exemption of employer provided medical care. . . . Each individual or family would, of course, be free to buy supplementary insurance, if it so desired (Emphasis added).

To put Friedman's policy recommendation in perspective, it may be noted that in 1990, at about the time Friedman formulated his recommendation, median pretax income in the United States was $29,943 for all households and $35,353 for "families," that is, for households with two or more members.[1] If we generously assume that Friedman meant to base the recommended deductible not on the sum of the family's income during the past two years but only on the average annual family income over the prior two years, then that deductible in 1990 would have been $10,500 per year for a family with median pretax income of $35,353. The outlays on medical care of a relatively healthy family probably would not have reached that deductible. A family stricken with serious illness

---

1. Alan Stockman, *Introduction to Microeconomics.* New York: The Dryden Press, 1996.

almost surely would have had to pay that much out of pocket before insurance coverage set in. In addition, of course, each family would have had to pay the premium for the catastrophic insurance policy.

Professor Friedman injected his editorial into the presidential election campaign of 1991–1992, in which health policy had moved to center stage. He acknowledged the contribution to his editorial by fellow Nobel Laureate economist Gary S. Becker of the University of Chicago and by economist Thomas Moore, Ph.D., formerly of President Reagan's Council of Economic Advisors and now at the Hoover Institute of Stanford University. In short, we may regard the editorial as a significant statement made by prominent American economists who sought to influence with their normative analysis both the election and the path of public health policy.

Surely neither Professor Friedman nor anyone else would assume for a moment that the distribution of health services in the United States, the distribution of the financial burden of illness, and the socio-demographic profile of health status would be the same under his proposal—including as it would the complete abolition of Medicare and Medicaid—as they would be in the presence of these programs or under yet another health reform proposal. His proposal might get us to the health economics analogue of Seattle (the rationing of health services and life-years by price and the individual's ability to pay) when, for all we know, the majority of Americans might well prefer the analogue of San Diego (access to health services by all members of society, on roughly equal terms, regardless of the individual's ability to pay for his or her own care). After all, none other than Republican President George Bush had flatly declared, in his State of the Union address in 1991, that "good health care is every American's right."

To suggest that a market-driven system such as that advocated by Professor Friedman would be more "efficient" than the current American health system with Medicare and Medicaid or, say, the British National Health Service or the Canadian health system, is an idiosyncratic, personal opinion that reflects a personally preferred distributional ethic for health services. It is not the product of "economic science" and certainly would not receive the endorsement even of the economics profession.[2] One simply cannot compare in terms of their relative "economic efficiency" health systems that espouse quite different social goals, any more than one can compare routes to Seattle and to San Diego in terms of their efficiency. None of this is to say, of course, that we ought not

---

2. Victor H. Fuchs, "Economics, Values and Health Care Reform," *American Economic Review* (86, March 1996): 1–24.

to search for relatively more efficient ways to reach the same social goals that are now being reached with the Medicare and Medicaid programs. It is simply to plead for a more thoughtful use of the much misused term "efficiency."

Well-trained economists know these *caveats*. We must therefore assume that economists who misuse the term "efficiency" in the context of policy analysis do so not as social scientists, but as political creatures who employ seemingly scientific methods to further personally preferred ideological ends. One finds that game played, of course, not only at one end of the ideological spectrum. One finds it played all along the entire ideological spectrum of our society. As I have warned countless Princeton students in several decades of teaching:

> When economists or other policy analysts lapse into their *normative* mode— when they pretend to be using scientific methods to suggest what *ought* to be done and what is "efficient" or is not—a red warning light should go on in your mind. Chances are that you are being addressed by someone playing politics in the guise of science or by someone insufficiently respectful of the limits of economics as a science.[3]

Given this perspective on our profession, I am delighted that colleague Thomas Rice has gone to the trouble of returning the spotlight to an intra-professional debate that, I had thought, had been decisively settled decades ago—by the then giants of our profession[4]—but whose outcome seems to have been all but forgotten or deliberately suppressed from memory by subsequent generations of economists. One must hope that this elegant book will quickly become a staple in undergraduate and graduate teaching, in economics as well as in schools of public health and health management. If nothing else, the book should trigger the revival of a philosophical debate that should be had anew by every generation of economists and policy analysts.

In this book, its author goes much beyond a mere dissection of the meaning of "efficiency." With meticulous and far-ranging scholarship he examines the entire battery of assumptions that must be valid and conditions that must be satisfied before an economist can, in good conscience, declare a so-called "market-driven" health system superior to alternative arrangements of producing and distributing health services.

Consider, for example, the seemingly innocuous proposition, so often employed by market devotees in health policy, that an individual's

3. In this connection, see Uwe E. Reinhardt, "Reflection on the Meaning of Efficiency: Can Efficiency Be Separated from Equity?" *Yale Law & Policy Review* (10, no. 2, 1992): 302–16.

4. See, for example, Francis M. Bator, "The Simple Economics of Welfare Economics," *American Economic Review* (72, August 1958): 351–79; and especially William J. Baumol, *Welfare Economics and the Theory of the State*. Cambridge, MA: Harvard University Press, 1969.

demand for care provides an acceptable yardstick of the social value of the care that individual receives. As Rice points out, the validity of that proposition presumes the absence of either "positive" or "negative externalities" in the use of health services—technical jargon for "compassion" and "envy," respectively. To assume away such externalities is dubious on its face. While one might work around the presence of compassion with an appeal to private, voluntary charity, how is one to incorporate into one's economic welfare calculus the presence of social envy—the fuel that literally drives economic progress in modern economies and that also severely constrains public health policy?

Then consider a baseline situation with a given distribution of care services among members of American society. Call it situation A. Now imagine the development of a highly effective but very expensive new medical technology that can extend substantially the life of critically ill patients but that will be made available only to wealthy patients who can pay for it. Call this situation B. If there were no negative externalities in the use of health services, the American public should judge situation B superior to situation A, because some people will be made better off by that technology and no one will receive less care than he or she previously had received. But can we be sure that the American public would, indeed, accept situation B with equanimity? For all we know, situation B might trigger social discord and make many Americans feel less well off.

In the same vein of reasoning, can the market devotees among economists blithely assume that Americans would accept with equanimity a health policy that lets transplantable organs be rationed strictly by the market—that is, by price and the individual patient's ability to pay? If not, then how can it be said that a market-driven health system, such as that proposed by Friedman and kindred spirits, is more "efficient" and "equitable" than some alternative algorithm for rationing care? With appeal to the so-called *Second Theorem of Welfare Economics*, economists sometimes try to circumvent this problem with the assertion that, in principle, the problem of the distribution of ability to pay among members of society can be separated from the problem of allocating resources efficiently by first letting the political process put in place an ethically acceptable distribution of purchasing power and then letting the free market allocate resources efficiently. As Kenneth J. Arrow, who offered that observation in his seminal paper on health economics was the first to acknowledge, however, in practice there is not available a mechanism of income redistribution that does not abet its own inefficiencies.[5] Furthermore, it can be doubted that there exists one single distribution of

---

5. Kenneth J. Arrow, "Uncertainty and the Welfare Economics of Medical Care," *American Economic Review* (78, December 1963): 942–73.

purchasing power that would satisfy the distributive ethic the American public may wish to impose on a variety of particular commodities.[6]

The critique offered in this valuable book, and yet other critiques of the literature advocating the "market" for health care,[7] should not be read as a broadside aimed at any proposal to engage the market approach in health policy, for the critique is not intended as such. There are many instances when market forces can, indeed, be constructively engaged in health services to achieve explicitly stated social goals. Rather, the book and other such critiques should be read as pleas that social goals not be posited inadvertently or surreptitiously in policy analysis, either through careless use of normative economic analysis or through deliberately mischievous use. It is difficult enough at times for economists to see through such tactics. It is well-nigh impossible for even highly educated laypersons to see through these tactics, let alone for the general public.

If one day the economics profession felt moved, through the good offices of its American Economic Association (AEA), to mimic the many other professions that profess allegiance to an explicit code of ethics, such a code would probably frown upon careless or duplicitous normative economic analysis. This book would be a good source for the development of such a code and the associated economic-practice guidelines. In any event, I hope that this book will be widely read and heeded, especially by the next cohorts in our profession.

Uwe E. Reinhardt, Ph.D.
James Madison Professor of Political Economy
Princeton University

6. Uwe E. Reinhardt, "Abstracting from Distributional Effects, This Policy is Efficient," in Morris L. Barer, Thomas E. Getzen, and Greg L. Stoddard, eds., *Health, Health Care and Health Economics*, New York: John Wiley & Sons, Ltd., 1979, pp. 1–53.

7. Morris L. Barer, Thomas E. Getzen, and Greg L. Stoddard, eds., *Health, Health Care and Health Economics*, 1979.

ACKNOWLEDGMENTS

UCH OF the research contained in this book was conducted while I was on a sabbatical from the University of California at Los Angeles. I would like to express my deep appreciation to a number of people for providing comments on the research itself or on the individual chapters: Henry Aaron, Ronald Andersen, William Comanor, Katherine Desmond, Robert Evans, Rashi Fein, Paul Feldstein, Susan Haber, Diana Hilberman, Donald Light, Harold Luft, David Mechanic, Glenn Melnick, Gavin Mooney, Joseph Newhouse, Mark Peterson, Uwe Reinhardt, John Roemer, Sally Stearns, Greg Stoddart, Deborah Stone, Pete Welch, and Joseph White. I would also like to thank Charles Doran and Karen Gorostieta for preparing the figures included in the book. It goes without saying that all conclusions, and any errors, are entirely my own.

1

INTRODUCTION

1.1 Why Should the Economics of Health Be Reconsidered?

I N RECENT years, there has been a surge of interest in reforming the organization and delivery of health systems by replacing government regulation with a reliance on market forces. Although much of the impetus has come from the United States, the phenomenon is worldwide. Spurred by ever-increasing costs, many analysts and policymakers have embraced the competitive market as the means of choice for reforming medical care systems. To a great extent, this belief stems from economic theory, which purports to show the superiority of markets over government regulation.

At the time of writing, there is indeed some evidence from the United States that increased competition in the health sector is controlling the rate of increase in costs. Between 1993 and 1995, for example, the percentage of workers covered by conventional insurance declined from 49 percent to 27 percent (Jensen et al. 1997). Over that same period, per capita national health expenditures rose by less than 6 percent annually—approximately the same amount as the economy as a whole, and far less than in previous years (Levit et al. 1996a; Levit, Lazenby, and Sivarajan 1996). In addition, various studies have shown that the geographic areas in which managed care penetration is highest have experienced the smallest increases in health costs (Zwanziger and Melnick 1996). Whether this indicates that the health services market in the United States is indeed operating in a more efficient manner than it used to be is less clear, however, as improved efficiency depends not only on costs, but also on what we are getting for the money.[1] More Americans are uninsured than previously, most likely in part because of additional competition among health insurers.[2] In addition, although the empirical evidence is still ambiguous, there is much concern now about how increased competition among providers and insurers has affected the quality of care provided.

The perceived success of this increasingly competitive marketplace in health services is perhaps emblematic of a larger trend in the United States, in which markets are viewed as "efficient" and government is viewed as "inefficient." As Robert Kuttner (1997) has written, "America . . . is in one of its cyclical romances with a utopian view of laissez-faire" (p. 4). This does not imply, either in the health sector or in the economy as a whole, that policymakers have eschewed government involvement. My concern, however, is that the trend is going in this direction, and that economic theory is used—inappropriately, it will be argued—in support of further market-based health policies.

Indeed, all health economists—even those favoring a more competitive marketplace—recognize that government needs to play a significant role in the health system. Much of the work in this area is based on the writings of Alain Enthoven, who has, over the last 20 years, advocated reliance on consumer choice and markets to improve the efficiency of health markets, with government playing two key roles: ensuring that competition is based on price rather than the selection of the healthiest patients, and providing subsidies to low-income persons.[3]

---

1. Alain Enthoven (1988) makes this point nicely, writing, "An efficient allocation of health care resources to and within the health care sector is one that minimizes the social cost of illness, including its treatment. This is achieved when the marginal dollar spent on health care produces the same value to society as the marginal dollar spent on education, defense, personal consumption, and other uses. Relevant costs include the suffering and inconvenience of patients, as well as the resources used in producing health care. This goal should not be confused with minimizing or containing health care expenditures. Policy makers focus much attention on the total amount of spending on health care services, often as a share of gross national product (GNP). But, a lower percentage of GNP spent on health care does not necessarily mean greater efficiency. If the reduced share of GNP is achieved by denial or postponement of services that consumers would value at more than their marginal cost, then efficiency is not achieved or enhanced by the cut in spending" (p. 11).

2. In the four-year period between 1991 and 1995, the percentage of nonelderly Americans who were uninsured rose from 16.0 to 17.4 percent (Employee Benefit Research Institute 1996).

3. Enthoven's earliest work in this area was published in *The New England Journal of Medicine* (Enthoven 1978), followed up by a book (Enthoven 1980). A significant revision of the proposal appears in Enthoven (1988) and Enthoven and Kronick (1989), in which "sponsors" such as large employers or consortia of small employers would serve as brokers for consumers who purchase health insurance.

The corollary to this viewpoint is that government *should* confine itself to only these two roles. Stated another way, competition should form the basis of policy in the health area, with government playing a subsidiary role of ensuring that markets operate fairly and that disadvantaged people are helped out. This conclusion, however, does not fall out of a careful review of economic theory as applied to health.

This book contends that one of the main reasons for the belief that market-based systems are superior stems from a misunderstanding of economic theory as it applies to health. As will be shown, such conclusions are based on a large set of assumptions that are not met, and cannot be met in the health sector. This is not to say that competitive approaches in this sector of the economy are inappropriate; rather, their efficacy depends on the particular circumstances of the policy being considered and the environment in which it is to be implemented. There is, however, no *a priori* reason to believe that such a system will operate more efficiently, or provide a higher level of social welfare, than alternative systems that are based instead on governmental financing and regulation. This argument is further bolstered by the fact that so many other developed countries have chosen to deviate from market-based health systems.

Although economists are aware that claims about the superiority of competitive approaches are based on fulfillment of a number of assumptions, a reading of the health literature indicates that there is little mention of either the large number of such assumptions, or of their importance. One should not put undue blame on health economists, however, because this problem pervades the entire economic discipline. In this regard, Lester Thurow (1983) has written that "every economist knows the dozens of restrictive assumptions . . . that are necessary to 'prove' that a free market is the best possible economic game, but they tend to be forgotten in the play of events" (p. 22).

Although the conclusion that competition will result in optimal economic outcomes is based on many assumptions, there is no generally agreed-upon list, as various economists have come up with different ones. The list presented below was drawn from several writers: Graaff (1971), Henderson and Quandt (1980), Mishan (1969a, 1969b), Nath (1969), Ng (1979), Rowley and Peacock (1975), and Sen (1982).

The book thus centers around a description, analysis, and application of these assumptions—and in particular, what happens if they are not met in markets for health services. The specific assumptions examined, along with the chapters in which they are analyzed, are shown in Table 1.1. (Some of these will not be self-explanatory to the noneconomist reader; they will be clarified in the specified chapters.) It is noteworthy that this is only a *partial* list of the assumptions on which the superiority of the competitive model is based. Other assumptions are not mentioned here either because they are essentially the same as those noted above, or because, in the author's opinion, the health economics profession has dealt with them adequately.[4]

1.2 Purpose of the Book

As the title suggests, the purpose of this book is to reconsider the economics of health. It does so by examining the assumptions on which the superiority of competitive approaches are based, and how, if they are not met, this affects health policy choices.

Although each chapter provides numerous applications, the book is really more about theory—both its use and its misuse. The book will attempt to show that *economic theory* provides no support for the belief that competition in healthcare will lead to superior social outcomes.

If one accepts the viewpoint that economic theory does not demonstrate the superiority of market forces in health, the obvious corollary is that all important questions must be answered empirically. And, to a large

---

4. One exception is the *theory of the second best*. Suppose that two or more of the assumptions in Table 1.1 are not met. It might seem reasonable to suppose that public policy should focus on trying to improve one of these particular market imperfections. This, however, is not necessarily the case. This theory states that if there are multiple factors that cause a market to deviate from the assumptions of market competition, then it is not necessarily appropriate to try to make the market more competitive in selected areas (Lipsey and Lancaster 1956–1957).

A hypothetical example in the health field might help clarify this. Suppose that two of the assumptions on which economic competition is based do not hold: there are few firms, which results in monopoly power; and consumer information is poor. The theory shows that more competition in one of these areas will not necessarily bring us any closer to an optimal state and, in fact, may have the opposite effect. If there are a limited number of firms, then better information about price might allow firms to set prices as in a cartel (Fielding and Rice 1993). Or if information were limited, then as the number of physicians in an area rose, it would become increasingly difficult for consumers to keep track of prices and reputation in the market. As a result, consumers might have to pay higher physician prices than they might otherwise (Satterthwaite 1979; Pauly and Satterthwaite 1981). Thus, even within the economic model, increased competition may not always be desirable.

Because so many assumptions of the competitive marketplace are not met in the health area, second-best considerations are pervasive. The most important one, perhaps, is the existence of health insurance itself. When consumers have health insurance, the price they pay out-of-pocket for services is less than the cost of providing the services. (In a competitive marketplace, prices and costs are equivalent in the long run.) The theory of the second best therefore tells us that *other* competitive policies are not necessarily optimal in the presence of health insurance.

One problem with using second-best considerations to critique competitive economic policies in the health area is that, realistically, none can pass a second-best test. As indicated, there are nearly always several aspects of a market that do not conform to the assumptions of competition. None of the arguments made in this book rely on second-best considerations. Readers wishing to pursue this topic should examine Robert Kuttner's (1997) book, *Everything for Sale: The Virtue and Limits of Markets*, for a detailed analysis of applying the theory of the second best to the health sector and to several other markets.

Table 1.1   Further Treatment of the Assumptions

Chapter 2: Market Competition
 1. There are no negative externalities of consumption.
 2. There are no positive externalities of consumption.
 3. Consumer tastes are predetermined.

Chapter 3: Demand Theory
 4. A person is the best judge of his or her own welfare.
 5. Consumers have sufficient information to make good choices.
 6. Consumers know, with certainty, the results of their consumption decisions.
 7. Individuals are rational.
 8. Individuals reveal their preferences through their actions.
 9. Social welfare is based solely on individual utilities, which in turn are based solely on the goods and services consumed.

Chapter 4: Supply Theory
 10. Supply and demand are independently determined.
 11. Firms do not have any monopoly power.
 12. Firms maximize profits.
 13. There are not increasing returns to scale.
 14. Production is independent of the distribution of wealth.

Chapter 5: Equity
 9. Social welfare is based solely on individual utilities, which in turn are based solely on the goods and services consumed.
 15. The distribution of wealth is approved of by society.

extent, that is exactly what most health economists and health services researchers are trying to do. I have few reservations about the kinds of research studies that are being conducted; rather, I am concerned that the work will suffer if researchers approach it with preconceived notions of what the results ought to be.

Economists often take the viewpoint that the way to test a theory—such as the purported advantages of market competition—is to see how well it predicts. This may work well when we are evaluating *positive* (i.e., factual) issues—say, the effect of a change in patient copayments on service utilization. It is less helpful in evaluating *normative* issues—those that involve the word "should."

The field of *welfare economics* deals in the latter kinds of issues—for example, *should* we rely on competitive policies in the health sector? In such instances, assessing how well the theory predicts does little good, because different analysts will disagree about which alternative state of the world is at a higher level of welfare. For example, if the United States were to adopt a Canadian-style system, there would likely be little agreement among health economists about whether the population was better off under the new system or the old one.

In this regard, Jan de V. Graaff (1971) has written,

> [W]elfare . . . is not an observable quantity like a market price or an item of personal consumption [so] it is exceedingly difficult to test a welfare proposition. . . . The consequence is that, whereas the normal way of testing a theory in positive economics is to test its conclusions, *the normal way of testing a welfare proposition is to test its assumptions*. . . . The result is that our assumptions must be scrutinized with care and thoroughness. Each must stand on its own two feet. We cannot afford to simplify much. (pp. 2–3, italics added)

Thus, it is vitally important that we get our theory right when applying economics to health—and the key to this is understanding the validity of the assumptions. If we do not, then we will blind ourselves to policy options that might actually be best at enhancing social welfare, many of which simply cannot be derived from the conventional economic model. One of the primary purposes of this book is to understand the implications that arise when many important assumptions that underlie the advantages of competition are not met in health services.

It is important also to set out what the book does *not* do. Some readers will be disappointed to see that, although the book critiques the competitive model, it does not explicitly offer an alternative in its place and compare the outcomes of each. To do so would be a hopeless undertaking. A small library could easily be filled with analyses of different countries' health policies—with little in the way of definitive conclusions. The book's goal is much more modest—to analyze what economic theory has to say about the role of competition in the health area. Ultimately, readers must draw their own conclusions about the most desirable sort of system, using not only theory but empirical observation as well.

This leads to a second limitation. Unlike some other health economics texts, this one does not attempt to summarize the empirical work in the field. As such, it is not designed to serve as a stand-alone textbook for courses in health economics or health policy. Rather, the book can be used as a supplementary textbook, in addition to one of the more traditional health economics texts, or along with a reader of classic or current economics journal articles.

This book is intended to serve several audiences, however, not just students. One of its primary audiences is health economics professionals in universities, research firms, management, and government. Although the book contains economic background that is hardly necessary for such an audience, the main theme is intended to strike a nerve, making readers realize that the case for relying on competitive markets in health does not arise from a careful reading of economic theory.

Finally, the book is also addressed to noneconomics professions. Because practitioners in these disciplines obviously tend to be less schooled in the details of economic analysis, they often have to take health economists at their word when the latter speak about the policy implications of economic analysis. (In this regard, Joan Robinson has been quoted as advising, "Study economics to avoid being deceived by economists" [Kuttner 1984, p. 1].) It is hoped that this book will help put those in other disciplines on a more level playing field when it comes to discussions of health policy.

1.3 Outline of the Book

The book is divided into six chapters. Chapters 2 through 4 deal with the three central themes of microeconomic theory: market competition, demand theory, and supply theory. The first 14 assumptions listed in Table 1.1 are analyzed in those chapters. Chapter 5 explores the final assumption, equity and redistribution, a topic of tremendous importance to policy but one that has been given insufficient attention by health economists. Chapter 6, the conclusion, offers some final thoughts concerning the role of competition in the health area.

Chapters 2 through 5 share a similar format. First, they present the traditional economic model, so that readers not familiar with intermediate microeconomics will find the remaining material accessible. Readers already familiar with the core concepts of microeconomic theory can skip these sections (Sections 2.1, 3.1, 4.1, and 5.1) and go directly to the two remaining parts of these chapters: problems with the traditional model (Sections 2.2, 3.2, 4.2, and 5.2), and implications for health policy (Sections 2.3, 3.3, 4.3, and 5.3).

2

MARKET COMPETITION

T HE ECONOMIES of nearly all developed countries are based on market competition. In health, the extent of reliance on private markets varies from country to country, with the United States generally being viewed as more "marketlike" than others. In recent years, however, there has been a movement in many (but not all) developed countries—not just the United States—to instill more market competition, and less government, into national health systems. This chapter, after presenting the reader with a good deal of background on competition, addresses whether economic theory provides a strong enough justification for enacting competitive policies in the health area.

Section 2.1 summarizes the traditional model of competition, including some of the standard tools of microeconomic analysis. Section 2.2 explores three of the most critical assumptions used in justifying the advantages of a competitive marketplace. Section 2.3 draws a number of implications for health policy.

2.1 The Traditional Economic Model

The field of microeconomics is devoted to the study of competition—mainly its virtues, but also some of its pitfalls. Although many of the techniques economists use are fairly new, the emphasis on competition—dating back to the writings of Adam Smith over 200 years ago—is not. Smith believed that people driven by their own economic interest in the marketplace are guided, by an "invisible hand," to act in a manner that ultimately is most beneficial to society at large.

The notion of competition is intuitively appealing. In a competitive market, people are allowed—but not compelled—to trade their stock of wealth, including their labor, if they find it beneficial to do so. Once everyone stops trading because no additional advantage is apparent, the market is in *equilibrium*. Such an outcome is desirable on two fronts: (1) people are making their own choices; and (2) by not engaging in any more trades, people *reveal themselves*[1] to be as satisfied with their economic lot as possible, given the resources with which they began.

This section outlines the economic theory of competition, what competition can and cannot achieve, and the assumptions on which this theory is based. It is divided into four subsections: Consumers, Producers, The Economy as a Whole, and Pareto Optimality and Social Welfare. The presentation is informal and brief, providing just enough information to support the remaining material in the book. Those familiar with standard microeconomic theory can proceed immediately to Section 2.2, and those seeking more detail on the material presented may wish to consult any of a number of microeconomics textbooks.[2]

2.1.1 Consumers

In consumer theory, people seek to maximize their *utility*, which is largely determined by the bundle of goods and services that they possess. To do so, they purchase their ideal bundle based on their desire or *taste* for alternative goods, and the prices of these alternatives, subject, of course, to how much income they have available to spend.

We will define U as the level of utility that a representative consumer receives from the consumption of alternative quantities of "n" different goods and services, indicated as X, Y, Z, and so on.

$$U = U(X, Y, Z, \ldots, n). \tag{2.1}$$

The utility obtained from consumption of one more unit of any good is called its *marginal utility*.

It is further assumed that consumers prefer more of a good to less of it, but that at some point, additional units of a particular good bring less utility than previous units; this is known as *diminishing marginal utility*. These concepts can be represented graphically by an *indifference curve*, which shows alternative combinations of two goods that result in the same level of utility. Indifference curves (examples of which are shown in Figure 2.1) tend to have a convex-to-the-origin shape because

---

1. Chapter 3, on the theory of demand, will focus on the concept of revealed preference.

2. There are many good introductory microeconomics textbooks. Parkin (1994) is an example. For a more advanced treatment of the subject, an excellent source is Henderson and Quandt (1980).

of diminishing marginal utility; once a person has a great deal of one good and little of another, that person has to receive a lot more of the former in order to give up even a little bit of the latter. The slope of the indifference curve is called the *marginal rate of substitution*. It is equal to the ratio of the marginal utilities of the two goods.[3]

To make this less abstract, Figure 2.1 shows only two goods that might appear in a consumer's utility function: visits to physicians (MDs) and visits to nurse practitioners (NPs). (For expository purposes, it is also helpful to assume that all of a person's money is spent on these two services.) The quantity of nurse practitioner visits appears on the horizontal axis, and the quantity of physician visits, on the vertical axis. The consumer is indifferent to all points on curve U_1, since by definition all points bring equal levels of satisfaction. As drawn, three NP visits and four MD visits (point *A*) are equal in desirability to five NP visits and three MD visits (point *B*). The person would be even happier to have more (for example, point *C* on curve U_2), but that would involve spending more money than he or she has available.

The choice of how much of each type of visit to purchase depends not only on how much the person wants each type, but also on the respective price. The way in which consumers maximize utility is to spend each successive dollar in a way that brings about the most utility. This means that when they have spent their last dollar, consumers will, across all of the goods in their utility function, have equalized the ratio of the marginal utilities (*MU*) with the price of the good. If we define P_m as the price of MD visits, and P_n as the price of NP visits, then, for a consumer who has maximized his or her utility,

$$MU_m/P_m = MU_n/P_n. \tag{2.2}$$

By cross-multiplying and rearranging the terms, this can also be written and thought of in another way, where the ratios of the marginal utilities are equal to the price ratios of the two goods:

$$MU_m/MU_n = P_m/P_n. \tag{2.3}$$

---

3. This can be demonstrated as follows. Along an indifference curve, the consumer's level of utility is constant. Thus, any movement along the curve (which defines the curve's slope) represents a change only in the way in which the consumer achieves a given level of utility. If he or she has more of Y and less of X, the gain in utility from the former must equal the loss in utility from the latter. Specifically,

$$(\Delta Y) \times (MU_Y) = (\Delta X) \times (MU_X).$$

Rearranging these terms, we find that the slope of the indifference curve ($\Delta Y/\Delta X$) equals the ratio of the marginal utilities of the two goods.

Figure 2.1 Consumer Indifference Curves

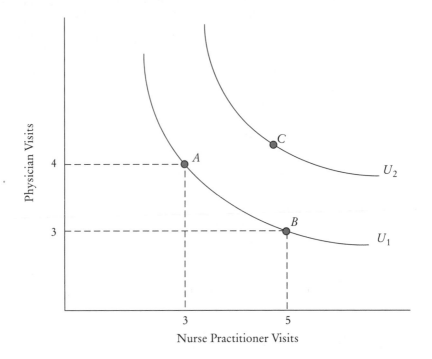

It is easy to see why a consumer must fulfill Equation 2.2 (and therefore also Equation 2.3) in order to maximize utility. Suppose that the equality is not met, because the marginal utility of each good equals 1 but the price of MD visits is $50 and the price of NP visits only $25. In this case, the consumer would not be in equilibrium but, rather, would find it beneficial to buy some more NP visits and fewer MD visits with his or her income. This will lower the marginal utility of NP visits, and raise it for MD visits. Only when both sides of Equation 2.2 (or 2.3) are equal will the consumer have nothing left to gain from trading.

This concept is illustrated in Figure 2.2. Here, the straight line is the consumer's *budget constraint*, which shows how many of each type of visit the consumer can purchase with a given income. Its slope is the price ratio between NP and MD visits; the point at which the line intersects each axis shows how many of each the consumer could buy by spending all income on that single service. At point A, the slope of the consumer's indifference curve is tangent to (i.e., has the same slope as) the budget constraint. In contrast, at point B they do not have the same slope, and the consumer is on an indifference curve that conveys less utility, U_0. By trading MD visits for NP visits, it is possible to move down the budget constraint to point *A*, and thereby to increase utility by moving to the higher indifference curve, U_1.

Although much of the above may seem fairly obvious, what is remarkable about the theory is that it shows that *everyone* will end up having the same marginal utilities for all goods and services. This is certainly clear mathematically; if everyone faces the same prices, the only way in which Equations 2.2 and 2.3 can hold is if everyone has the same marginal utilities. How can that be achieved? Suppose a person really prefers NP visits and only wants an occasional MD visit. At the prevailing price ratio, the person will purchase far more NP visits. But at some point, that person will have so many NP visits, and so few MD visits, that his or her marginal utility for MD visits—the satisfaction brought about by consumption of the last one—will finally fall to that of NP visits.

In summary, consumer theory tells us something very important. It concludes that people, taking into account their own preferences and market prices, can make choices that will make them best off. When they have done as well as they can do, given their resources, they stop trading, presumably to enjoy the mix of goods that they have acquired. These

Figure 2.2 The Consumer "Optimum"

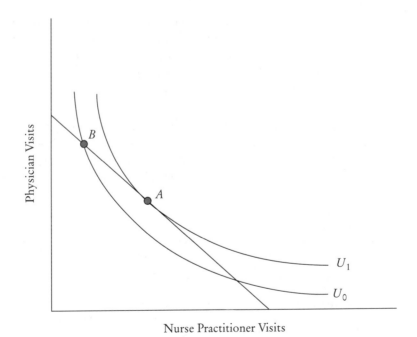

Nurse Practitioner Visits

are strong conclusions; much of Chapters 2 and 3 will be devoted to examining and critiquing the assumptions on which they are based.

2.1.2 Producers

In production theory, firms seek to maximize profits in a way analogous to the way in which consumers attempt to maximize utility. To do so, they purchase inputs and transform them into outputs through the application of some sort of technology. This process is represented through a *production function*.

We will use one of the goods discussed above, MD visits, but this time will examine how it is produced by a firm. Assume that there are "m" ($a, b, \ldots, m$) inputs that are used in producing these visits through a production process "f." The production function therefore takes the form,

$$\text{Visits} = f(a, b, \ldots, m). \tag{2.4}$$

The two most important classes of inputs are labor and capital.

Again, parallel to consumer theory, we assume that, given a fixed level of the other inputs, at some point additional units of a particular input will be less and less productive, a concept called *diminishing marginal productivity*. These concepts can be represented graphically by *isoquants*, as shown in Figure 2.3. Quantities of each of two inputs, a and b, are represented on the two axes; the isoquant labeled "Visits" shows the alternative quantity of inputs required to produce a certain number of visits. The other isoquant indicates the inputs necessary for producing "More Visits." The slope of an isoquant is called the *marginal rate of technical substitution* and is equal to the ratios of the marginal productivities of each input.[4]

If, given the state of technology, a firm produces as much output as possible with a given amount of inputs, production is known to be *technically efficient*. That does not necessarily mean, however, that it is *economically efficient*; for economic efficiency, it is also necessary

---

4. This can be demonstrated as follows. Along an isoquant, the output level is constant. Thus, any movement along the curve (which defines the curve's slope) represents a change only in the way in which the inputs are combined to achieve a given level of output. If we use more of input a and less of input b in producing X, the total amount of X produced cannot change. Specifically,

$$(\Delta a) \times (MP_a) = (\Delta b) \times (MP_b),$$

where MP is the marginal product (i.e., the amount produced from) the last unit of that input. Rearranging these terms, we find that the slope of the isoquant curve ($\Delta b / \Delta a$) equals the ratio of the marginal products of the two inputs.

Figure 2.3 Producer Isoquants

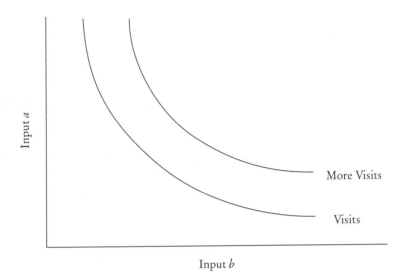

to use the mix of inputs that incurs the least costs. Only then can a firm maximize its profits. To produce in an economically efficient manner, a firm must therefore take into account the prices of alternative inputs, which are shown by an *isocost* line in Figure 2.4. The isocost line indicates the price ratio of the two inputs. As in the case of consumer theory, the firm achieves its goal—here, profit maximization—at point *A*, where the isocost and isoquant lines are tangent. At point *B*, where the lines are not tangent, the production process would be economically inefficient. Although *B* is on an isoquant, that isoquant is associated with fewer visits being produced, as indicated by the dashed line.

Suppose we have two inputs, labor (L) and capital (K), with their respective prices defined as the wage rate (w) and the rate of return on capital (r). A firm will thus maximize profits in the following situation:

$$MP_L/P_L = MP_K/P_K. \tag{2.5}$$

By cross-multiplying and rearranging the terms, this can also be written in another way, where the ratios of the marginal products of the two inputs are equal to their price ratios,

$$MP_L/MP_K = P_L/P_K. \tag{2.6}$$

To see why a firm must fulfill Equation 2.5 (or 2.6) to maximize profits, imagine that the equality is not met; the marginal productivity of

Figure 2.4 The Producer "Optimum"

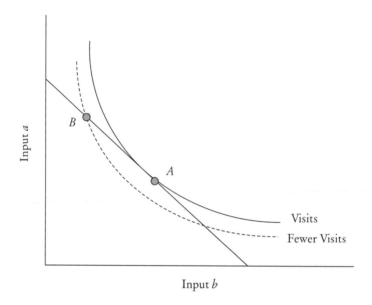

each input equals 1, but the price of labor is $10 and the price of capital is $5. In such a situation, the firm will find it beneficial to buy or use more capital and less labor. Eventually, capital will become less productive due to diminishing marginal productivity. Only when both sides of Equation 2.5 (or 2.6) are equal will the firm have no economic reason to change the ratio of inputs that it uses. And since all firms face the same input prices, they will all have the same ratio of marginal productivities.

After choosing the economically efficient mix of inputs, firms must decide how much output to produce and the price for which they will sell their output. In a competitive market, in which the products of alternative firms are indistinguishable, there really is no choice regarding price: a firm will lose its market if it charges more than the going price, and it will not maximize profits if it charges less. The rule of thumb for choosing the quantity to produce is to equate the *marginal cost* (MC) of production—that is, the cost of producing the last good—to the market price that can be obtained by selling the good. This is shown as point A in Figure 2.5, with a corresponding quantity Q produced at price P. In the figure, the firm faces a fixed or horizontal market price for selling the good, but the

Figure 2.5 How Competitive Firms Choose Output Levels

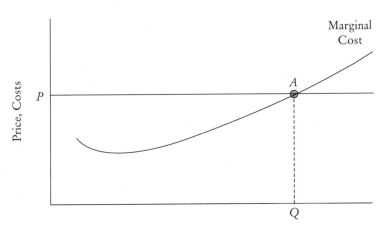

marginal cost curve slopes upward, reflecting the likelihood that it will cost more and more to produce successive units of output.[5]

The profit motive drives firms' decisions. If firms are able to make profits because, say, consumers suddenly want more of a particular product or because a new technology makes its production cheaper, existing firms will expand their output and/or other firms will enter the market, either of which will bring down the market price and eventually make profits fall back to a *normal*[6] rate of return. If firms incur losses, perhaps due to depressed consumer demand, they will cut back on production and/or some will leave the market, again until a normal rate of profits returns.

All of the above refers to *short-run* firm decisions. This period of time varies from industry to industry. The short run is a period in which the firm cannot vary its capital stock, but can vary labor inputs. In the long run, the firm can vary all of its inputs. The key long-run decision that a firm must make is how much capital to purchase, and this depends, to a large degree, on its anticipation of the size of its market.

---

5. As discussed below, the analysis being described here is called the short run, which is defined as the period of time over which capital inputs are fixed. Thus, to produce more output, the only choice is to use more labor. Eventually, however, too many laborers "crowd" the fixed amount of capital, making each successive laborer less productive. This will, in turn, raise the cost of production; thus, the marginal cost curve will slope upward.

6. A normal rate of return can be viewed as the rate of return on money invested in a different endeavor that has similar risk. If a firm does not earn at least a normal rate of return in an industry, it would do better to shut down and invest resources elsewhere.

In summary, production theory tells us that firms will seek to use their inputs most efficiently, and make their output choices, in a way that maximizes their profits. But in doing so, they also serve certain social purposes by (1) not wasting inputs, and (2) only producing those goods and services that consumers demand. Next, we describe the interaction of the many consumers and products that make up the economy as a whole.

2.1.3 The Economy as a Whole

Up until now, we have considered the consumer and producer sectors of the economy separately. This is inadequate, however, because the goods and services consumed in an economy must also be the exact ones that are produced, and consumers must purchase them at the same price for which firms sell them. Furthermore, changes in the market for a particular good or service may affect other markets as well. Viewing the consumption or production of a single good is called *partial equilibrium analysis*, while considering the economy as a whole is known as *general equilibrium analysis*.

Figure 2.6 illustrates a *production possibility frontier* (PPF), which shows the amount of each of two goods (NP visits and MD visits) that can be produced, given the amount of inputs that are available to the economy. Producing more MD visits will use scarce inputs that will no longer be available to produce NP visits. Hence, fewer NP visits will be produced. The slope of the PPF is called the *marginal rate of transformation*; it indicates how much of one good or service must be sacrificed to produce an extra unit of the other. The concave-to-the-origin shape indicates that costs increase as we shift production from one type of visit to the other. We will assume that our competitive market produces at point *A* on the PPF, that is, ten NP visits and eight MD visits.

Figure 2.7 uses the same information to produce an *Edgeworth Box*, named for economist Francis Edgeworth. It shows how the output at point *A* can be divided between two consumers, Paul and Jane. Paul's allotment of both types of visits is shown in the normal fashion; at point *A*, he has about six (of the ten) NP visits and five (of the eight) MD visits. Jane's allotment, on the other hand, is depicted by looking in the opposite direction (downward for MD visits and from right to left for NP visits). She therefore gets the remaining four NP visits and three MD visits.

The figure also shows various sets of indifference curves for each consumer. We saw earlier that equilibrium can occur only when consumers have the same marginal rate of substitution, which occurs where their indifference curves are tangent, along the *contract curve O–A*.

Figure 2.6   Production Possibility Frontier

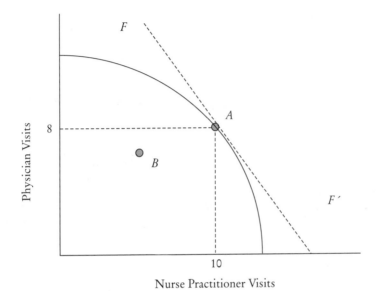

Nurse Practitioner Visits

General equilibrium analysis shows that, for production and exchange to be efficient, consumers' marginal rates of substitution must be equal to the economy's marginal rate of transformation. That is, the slope of the consumers' indifference curves at equilibrium, indicated by the line *I–I'*, must be equal to the slope of the PPF at point *A*, indicated by the line *F–F'* in Figure 2.6.

Why must this be the case? Suppose that the marginal rate of substitution between NP and MD visits is 1, but the marginal rate of transformation is 2. If Jane, one of our consumers, reduces her consumption of MD visits by one, she needs to get one more NP visit to be indifferent. But by producing one less MD visit, the economy would be able to produce two more NP visits. That leaves an extra NP visit available that could be given to Paul or to Jane. Thus, if the marginal rates of substitution and transformation are not equal, the economy is not in equilibrium, because it is possible to make one person better off without making another worse off.

2.1.4 Pareto Optimality and Social Welfare

When the consumption and production markets are in equilibrium, and when consumers' rates of indifference are equal to the economy's ability to transform one good into the others, we are in a position called *Pareto*

Figure 2.7   Edgeworth Box

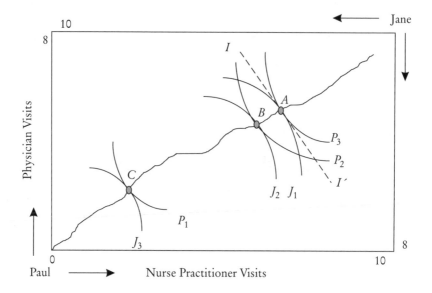

optimality, named after economist Vilfredo Pareto. In an economy that is in a Pareto-optimal state, it is impossible to make someone better off (that is, increase that person's welfare) without making someone else worse off. Under such a situation, the economy has reached a state of *allocative efficiency*, although as we shall see in the next section, this rests on a number of assumptions.

How does an economy reach Pareto optimality? Economists have shown that if certain conditions are met, a free or competitive market, operating on its own, will reach a *competitive equilibrium* that is Pareto optimal. Thus, allowing competition to occur will result in a situation where it is impossible to make someone better off without making someone else worse off.

The concept of Pareto optimality, although useful from a theoretical standpoint, is rather weak from a policy standpoint: it provides little guidance. This is because of the difficulty of imagining even a single public policy that would make some people better off without making another person or persons worse off. Suppose, for example, that the government chooses to subsidize immunizations against chickenpox. Although seemingly benign, such a policy would make worse off a taxpayer with no children who had already had the disease as a child; there would be costs to this person but no benefits.[7]

---

7. Of course, if this person were benevolent, he or she might find the policy desirable. This issue is taken up later, where we discuss positive externalities of consumption.

If there are winners and losers associated with all policies, then deciding between policies to enact involves a value judgment, namely, who should benefit and who should lose? Making such a determination is beyond the realm of economic analysis. Consequently, over the years, economists have tried to develop tools to make it easier for them to make policy recommendations that are not value-laden. However, the two main examples of this—classical utilitarianism[8] and the Kaldor-Hicks criterion[9]—have been strongly refuted in the economics literature.

It is important to recognize that market competition in general, and Pareto optimality in particular, do not address issues of equity or the desirability of the distribution of income that results from the workings of a competitive economy. Thus, a competitive equilibrium can occur in which one person has nearly all of the output, and another has almost none. In fact, this can easily occur if the former person begins with the vast majority of initial wealth or inputs. Amartya Sen (1970) makes this point graphically:

> An economy can be [Pareto] optimal . . . even when some people are rolling in luxury and others are near starvation as long as the starvers cannot be made better off without cutting into the pleasures of the rich. If preventing the burning of Rome would have made Emperor Nero feel worse off, then letting him burn Rome would have been Pareto-optimal. In short, a society or an economy can be Pareto-optimal and still be perfectly disgusting. (p. 22)

Although it might seem desirable to transfer wealth from the rich person to the poor person, doing so cannot be viewed as improving the economy from a Paretian viewpoint, because the change will involve making the rich person worse off. Under the traditional economic model, competition is designed to enhance efficiency; it does not necessarily improve equity.

This point is critical because members of society do care about equity.[10] This means that a Pareto-optimal competitive equilibrium does not necessarily make society best off. In fact, it is highly plausible that a society will be better off with an inefficient use of resources (that is, at point *B* inside the PPF in Figure 2.6) *and* a desirable distribution of income, than it would be at point *A* with a poor distribution.

---

8. Utilitarianism is discussed at greater length in Sections 3.1 and 5.2.

9. The Kaldor-Hicks criterion states that an economic change is desirable if the "winners" can compensate the "losers" to get the latter to agree to the change—but they do not have to follow through with the compensation!

10. Blendon et al. (1994) report on U.S. survey results indicating a strong moral commitment to the uninsured. At the same time, only 23 percent of Americans agreed with the statement, "It is the responsibility of the government to take care of very poor people who can't take care of themselves"; this compares to 50 percent of Germans, 56 percent of Polish, 62 percent of British and French, 66 percent of Italians, and 71 percent of Spanish people (Blendon et al. 1995a).

Thus, it is natural to ask whether some Pareto-optimal points (i.e., points on the contract curve O–A in Figure 2.7) are socially more desirable than others. To figure this out, it is necessary to make value judgments about how each person's utility affects society's total welfare. This is often illustrated by a *social welfare function*, as shown in Equation 2.7,

$$W = W(U_1, U_2, \ldots, U_n), \tag{2.7}$$

where W is society's total welfare, U indicates individual utility levels, and the subscripts represent each person in the population.

Coming up with society's social welfare function is no easy task. It could be imposed by a dictator, of course, but if one prefers more democratic means, a problem arises. The problem, which is proved in Kenneth Arrow's (1963a) *Possibility Theorem*, is that any method of aggregating individual preferences into a social welfare function violates at least one reasonable and desirable ethical condition. Thus, it turns out to be quite hard to come up with a desirable consensus on how to confront distributional issues, an issue to which we will return in Chapter 5.

2.2 Problems with the Traditional Model

Given that the above "textbook" model of competition forms the basis of economic training at both the undergraduate and graduate levels, it would appear that the traditional economic model of competition has a strong grip on economists in general. Only one study, however, has documented the views of health economists on issues such as the desirability of market competition in the health area. This was from a 1989 mailed survey of almost 300 individuals in the United States and Canada who consider themselves to be health economists, the results of which were summarized by Roger Feldman and Michael Morrisey (1990).

One of the questions asked in this survey was whether the respondent believed that the "competitive model cannot apply" to health. Interestingly, respondents were evenly divided on this question; half thought the model could apply, and half did not. More noteworthy, perhaps, were some of the response patterns to the question. Two-thirds of respondents who received their doctoral degrees from top economics departments thought that the competitive model could apply, versus 53 percent with degrees from other economics departments. Few of those who received their training in noneconomics departments believed that the competitive model could apply to the health system. Other patterns showed that younger respondents were more likely to believe in the competitive model, as were U.S. (versus Canadian) respondents.

In another survey that, among other things, sought to find out whether all health economists think alike, Victor Fuchs (1996) found a great deal of agreement on so-called positive (factual) issues, but very little on normative (opinion) ones[11]—which would presumably include whether health economists believe that the competitive model can apply to the health market.

The remainder of this section examines three reasons why the use of market competition may not lead to the highest level of social welfare. Section 2.3 will then provide some applications to health.

This critique of the competitive model is divided into three parts, in accordance with the first three of the assumptions listed in Table 1.1:

Assumption 1. There are no negative externalities of consumption.

Assumption 2. There are no positive externalities of consumption.

Assumption 3. Consumer tastes are predetermined.

One of the key assumptions with regard to the advantages of competition is that there are no externalities of consumption—or alternatively, that any such externalities are explicitly dealt with through public policy. A consumption externality exists when one person's consumption of a good or service has an effect on the utility of another person. There are positive and negative externalities of consumption. With a positive externality, one person's consumption of a good raises the utility of another person. With a negative externality, the consumption lowers another person's utility.

Certain consumption externalities have received much attention from health economists. Perhaps the classic example of a positive externality of consumption in all of economics, not just health, is immunizations. If I receive an immunization, I will not be the only beneficiary because my immunization also makes it less likely that others will get the disease, since they cannot catch it from me. But because, in a competitive market, an individual bears the full cost of the immunization, too few immunizations will be purchased. Recall that consumers purchase goods

---

11. For example, almost all health economists disagreed with the positive statements: that "the high cost of health care in the United States makes U.S. firms substantially less competitive in the global economy"; "widespread use of currently available screening and other diagnostic techniques would result in a significant reduction in health care expenditures 5 years from now"; and "differential access to medical care across socioeconomic groups is the primary reason for differential health status among these groups." However, opinions about normative issues were much less uniform. For example, about half of the health economists agreed with the statement, "the U.S. should seek universal coverage through a broad-based tax with implicit subsidies for the poor and the sick." Of the 13 normative questions, 11 of them showed substantial differences of opinion, which I define as between 25 percent and 75 percent of respondents agreeing with the statements. This was true of only one of the seven positive statements (Fuchs 1996).

until the ratio of the marginal utility of each to its price is equal across all goods (Equation 2.2). When there is a positive consumption externality, society's marginal utility is greater than that of the individual, so that consumers, acting on their own, will not purchase a large enough quantity of such goods.

A parallel argument can be made about negative externalities such as smoking. If my smoking lowers your utility, then society's marginal utility from my smoking will be lower than my own. Hence, in making consumption decisions through equalizing the marginal utility and prices of all goods, people will smoke more than is in society's best interest.

The existence of important externalities like these means that the operation of a competitive market, by itself, will not result in a socially optimal outcome. One possible way to improve matters is through government intervention. In the case of a positive externality like immunizations, government can subsidize their provision, even providing them free of charge. By funding such a program through taxes, most tax-payers would help contribute, which would seem desirable since so many people are benefiting. Dealing with a negative consumption externality like smoking is somewhat more problematic. Although it is easy to tax smokers by enacting special taxes on the production of cigarettes, it is much harder to ensure that this revenue is disbursed to those who are most affected by smoking. As a result, governmental bodies in the United States have taken an additional route by prohibiting smoking from many public places.

In this section we will deal with two different types of consumption externality (one negative and one positive) that have received far less consideration from economists—and which, perhaps not coincidentally, cannot be easily rectified through simple taxes and subsidies. The negative consumption externality is concern about status and rank; the positive one is concern about the well-being of others. We will argue below that it is quite plausible that most people are simultaneously subject to both of these mental traits.

2.2.1 Negative Externality: Concern about Status

In considering the problem to be examined in this section, recall Equation 2.1, in which a consumer's utility (U) was assumed to depend on the various quantities of the goods and services ($X, Y, Z, \ldots, n$) possessed:

$$U = f(X, Y, Z \ldots, n). \tag{2.1}$$

It was also assumed that having more of each good was better.

What is more important is what is *not* in the equation; *there is no consideration given to how one's bundle of goods and services compares to, and affects or is affected by, the bundles of goods and services that other people possess.*

Let us for a moment suppose that a person's utility function is more complicated; it depends not only on the quantity of goods (X, Y, Z) a person has, but also on how this compares to how much other people have, on average (as indicated by the bars above the letters). We will denote this as follows:

$$U = f\left(X, Y, Z, \frac{X}{\overline{X}}, \frac{Y}{\overline{Y}}, \frac{Z}{\overline{Z}}\right). \tag{2.8}$$

This states that a person's utility is determined not only by what he or she has, but by how this compares to the average of the population. (A more realistic formulation might have as a comparison those people with whom a person has most contact, or those in the same social class.)

Alternatively, one could even imagine a utility function where *only* one's position relative to others matters,[12] as shown in Equation 2.9,

$$U = f\left(\frac{X}{\overline{X}}, \frac{Y}{\overline{Y}}, \frac{Z}{\overline{Z}}\right). \tag{2.9}$$

A few well-known economists have, over the years, noted the substantial implications for the competitive model if one believes that relative as well as absolute wealth matters. Lord (Lionel) Robbins (1984) wrote that:

> If the remaining groups regard their position relatively, they may well argue that the spectacle of such improvement elsewhere is a detriment to their satisfaction. This is not a niggling point: a relative improvement in the position of certain groups *pari passu* with an absolute improvement in the position of the rest of the community has often been a feature of economic history; and we know that has not been regarded by all as either ethically or politically desirable. (pp. xxii–xxiii)

Similarly, Francis Bator (1958) states that

> [M]arket efficiency is neither sufficient nor necessary for market institutions to be the "preferred" mode of social organization. . . . If, e.g., people are sensitive not only to their own jobs but to other people's as well, or more generally, if such things as relative status, power, and the like, matter, the injunction to maximize output, to hug the production-possibility frontier, can hardly be assumed "neutral," and points on the utility frontier may associate with points inside the production frontier. (p. 378)

---

12. Yet another possibility is that one's absolute wealth matters up to a subsistence level, after which only relative wealth matters.

We therefore need to ask which of the above equations is the best representation of people's actual behavior? Intuition tells us that Equation 2.1 is implausible if not downright wrong. This equation implies that people are indifferent about their rank in society, have no concern about status, and do not worry about "keeping up with the Joneses." Rather, all that they care about is what they themselves have, irrespective of whether this is more or less, better or worse, than others with whom they have contact.

If this were true, then:

- How can one account for much if not most advertising, which tries to convey how favorably one will be viewed by others if one owns a particular car, wears a particular type of jeans, or drinks a particular brand of beer?

- How can one account for people's concern about their coworkers' salaries?

- How can one account for the following example, similar to one suggested by Robert Frank (1985): Give each of two siblings one piece of candy, and both children will be happy. But give two pieces to one child and three to another, and the child who receives the smaller share will be less happy than if each received only one. (A little introspection is likely to reveal that adults tend to react in the same manner.)

In this regard, A. C. Pigou (1932), one of the founders of modern economics, quotes and affirms John Stuart Mill's statement that "Men do not desire to be *rich*, but to be richer than other men" (p. 90). (In a lighter vein, Frank [1985] notes that "H. L. Mencken once defined wealth as any income that is at least one hundred dollars more a year than the income of one's wife's sister's husband" [p. 5].) Lester Thurow (1980) has stated that, once incomes exceed the subsistence level, "individual perceptions of the adequacy of their economic performance depend almost solely on relative as opposed to absolute position" (p. 18).

It is perhaps not unnatural to think that, while other people may behave in this manner, you and I are above such petty concerns about rank and status. Such a viewpoint is hard to hold, however, after giving consideration to the following thought experiment provided by Frank (1985):

In this experiment you are to imagine yourself in the following situation: As a high-income resident of the United States, you are suddenly confronted with an opportunity to be transported to a much richer planet. The trip will be free of charge, but with no option of return. You are a genuine standout here on Earth. You earn $100,000 per year and live in a tastefully decorated home in a quiet, fashionable neighborhood. Your children are enrolled in the best schools and are very popular among their classmates. You are happily married to a person you hold in high esteem, who regards you likewise. You are a person of integrity, a highly respected expert in your profession, and are in good health. You enjoy peace of mind and the admiration and affection of a large group of friends, who regard you as one of the most charming and caring people they know.

On the new planet your income would be $1,000,000 per year. But instead of being near the top of the income scale as you are here, you would be at the bottom. The home you would be able to afford there is much larger and better appointed than the one you live in here. Yet it is located in a marginal neighborhood, one that people urge their children not to venture into. You would pursue the same occupation there as you do here. But the people on the new planet are so skilled that they regard your profession in the way we think of repetitive, assembly tasks here. The schools your children would go to there compare very favorably with the ones they go to here, but among schools on the new planet they are thought to be ill-equipped and poorly staffed. Although your children will amass more knowledge in those schools than they do in the ones here, they will struggle there on the academic borderline, instead of bringing home A's as they do here. Although your children are much sought after by their classmates here, you will discover on the new planet that most parents attempt to steer their children to more suitable playmates. You will recount the same anecdotes there as you do here, but your friends there will regard them as simple and boring, instead of clever and erudite as your friends here regard them. Although your spouse will love you equally there as here, you know that, once there, he or she cannot fail to notice how the achievements of others surpass your own. (pp. 116–17)

Frank contends that you would be willing to give up $900,000 in income in order to retain your current status; it is hard to disagree.

The discussion up until this point has been intuitive, so it is natural to ask whether there is any evidence supporting the superiority of Equation 2.8 or 2.9 over Equation 2.1. Two classic studies are relevant here. James Duesenberry (1952) developed the *relative income hypothesis*. Under this hypothesis, people's drive for self-esteem makes them wish to emulate the consumption habits of those who are on a higher socioeconomic rung of the ladder; he states that "this drive operates through inferiority feelings aroused by unfavorable comparisons between living standards" and is heightened with more frequent contact between "the quality of the goods he uses with those used by others" (p. 31). The theory predicts that people with lower incomes will save a smaller proportion of their income because they will have more frequent contact with those in the economic class just above them, whose consumption patterns they will mimic. This prediction has been verified repeatedly through empirical studies.

Table 2.1 Percentage Not Very Happy in Lowest and Highest Status Groups, Seven Countries, 1965

		Lowest Status Group		Highest Status Group		
Country	Number of Groups	Designation	N.V.H.[a] (%)	Designation	N.V.H.[a] (%)	*N*
Great Britain	3	Very poor	19	Upper, upper middle, middle	4	1,179
West Germany	3	Lower middle, lower	19	Upper, upper middle	7	1,255
Thailand	2	Lower, middle	15	Middle, upper	6	500
Philippines	2	Lower middle, lower	15	Upper, upper middle	5	500
Malaysia	2	Lower, middle	20	Middle, upper	10	502
France	3	Lower	27	Upper	6	1,228
Italy	3	Lower middle, lower	42	Upper, upper middle	10	1,166

[a] N.V.H. = Not very happy.
Source: Easterlin, R. 1974. *Nations and Households in Economic Growth: Essays in Honor of Moses Abramovitz*, edited by P. A. David and M. W. Reder, p. 101. New York: Academic Press.

Further evidence is provided in Richard Easterlin's (1974) classic study of human happiness in 14 countries, some of the results of which are reproduced in Tables 2.1 and 2.2 and Figure 2.8. He found that in a given country at a given time, wealthier people tend to be happier than poorer people (Table 2.1). However, in a given country over time, happiness levels are surprisingly constant even in the wake of rising real incomes. (Table 2.2 shows data from the United States.) Furthermore, average levels of happiness are fairly constant across countries; people in poor countries and wealthy countries claim to be about equally happy (Figure 2.8). The only way such findings can be reconciled is if it is relative wealth rather than absolute wealth that matters. From this, Easterlin concludes:

> [T]here is a "consumption norm" which exists in a given society at a given time, and which enters into the reference standard of virtually everyone. This provides a common point of reference in self-appraisals of well-being, leading those below the norm to feel less happy and those above the norm, more happy. Over time, this norm tends to rise with the general level of consumption. . . . (pp. 112–13)

Curiously, the study seems to provide evidence that Equation 2.9 may be more in keeping with actual human behavior than Equation 2.8; in Equation 2.9, *only* one's relative standing matters. This is consistent with Easterlin's findings that wealthy people are about equally happy across countries, whether the countries are richer or poorer, and that poor people are about equally happy across countries. If one's absolute

Table 2.2 Percent Distribution of Population by Happiness, United States, 1946–1970

Date	Very Happy	Fairly Happy	Not Very Happy	Other	N
Apr. 1946	39	50	10	1	3,151
Dec. 1947	42	47	10	1	1,434
Aug. 1948	43	43	11	2	1,596
Nov. 1952	47	43	9	1	3,003
Sept. 1956	53	41	5	1	1,979
Sept. 1956	52	42	5	1	2,207
Mar. 1957	53	43	3	1	1,627
July 1963	47	48	5	1	3,668
Oct. 1966	49	46	4	2	3,531
Dec. 1970	43	48	6	3	1,517

Source: Easterlin, R. 1974. *Nations and Households in Economic Growth: Essays in Honor of Moses Abramovitz*, edited by P. A. David and M. W. Reder, p. 109. New York: Academic Press.

possessions mattered as well, one would expect to see people in wealthy countries exhibit a greater level of happiness than those of similar rank in poor countries. In addition, over times of rising real income, people in a particular country should also be happier.

One has to be careful not to infer too much from cross-national comparisons of happiness, mainly because factors other than economic status are likely to play different roles in the happiness levels of people from different countries.[13] Even so, accepting Equation 2.9, where the overriding determinant of happiness is one's relative rather than absolute standing, might seem a little hard. It implies that if I had more, but my relative standing remained the same, I would be no happier. This clearly contradicts the meaning of the indifference curves shown in Figure 2.1, in which it was assumed that more of each good would put a person at a higher level of utility.

Although Easterlin's study does not explicitly attempt to refute the concept of the indifference curve, his research also helps provide an understanding of why people might behave in a way that is so contradictory to traditional economic theory. He reports the results of a study by Hadley Cantril (1965) based on 1960s surveys of individuals living in the United States and India, concerning what makes them happy. Following are several quotations that strongly indicate that the things that make people happy vary dramatically with their circumstances:

---

13. Easterlin does demonstrate, however, that the concept of happiness translates consistently into the different languages of different countries. He therefore argues that his findings are not the result of the vagaries of language.

Figure 2.8 Personal Happiness Rating and GNP per Capita, 1960

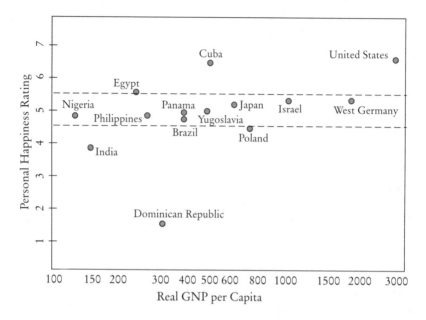

Source: Easterlin, R. 1974. *Nations and Households in Economic Growth: Essays in Honor of Moses Abramovitz*, edited by P. A. David and M. W. Reder, p. 106. New York: Academic Press.

India. I want a son and a piece of land since I am now working on land owned by other people. I would like to construct a house of my own and have a cow for milk and ghee. I would also like to buy some better clothing for my wife. If I could do this then I would be happy. [35-year-old man, illiterate, agricultural laborer, income about $10 a month]

India. I wish for an increase in my wages because with my meager salary I cannot afford to buy decent food for my family. If the food and clothing problems were solved, then I would feel at home and be satisfied. Also if my wife were able to work the two of us could then feed the family and I am sure would have a happy life and our worries would be over. [35-year-old sweeper, monthly income around $13]

India. I should like to have tap water and a water supply in my house. It would be able to have electricity. My husband's wages must be increased if our children are to get an education and our daughter is to be married. [45-year-old housewife, family income about $80 a month]

India. I hope in the future I will not get any disease. Now I am coughing. I also hope I can purchase a bicycle. I hope my children will study well and that

I can provide them with an education. I also would sometime like to own a fan and maybe a radio. [45-year-old skilled worker earning $30 a month]

U.S.: If I could earn more money I would be able to buy our own home and have more luxury around us, like better furniture, a new car, and more vacations. [27-year-old skilled worker]

U.S.: I would like a reasonable enough income to maintain a house, have a new car, have a boat, and send my four children to private schools. [34-year-old laboratory technician]

U.S.: I would like a new car. I wish all my bills were paid and I had more money for myself. I would like to play more golf and to hunt more than I do. I would like to have more time to do the things I want to and to entertain my friends. [24-year-old bus driver]

U.S.: Materially speaking, I would like to provide my family with an income to allow them to live well—to have the proper recreation, to go camping, to have music and dancing lessons for the children, and to have family trips. I wish we could belong to a country club and do more entertaining. We just bought a new home and expect to be perfectly satisfied with it for a number of years. [28-year-old lawyer] (Cantril 1965, as quoted in Easterlin 1974, 114–15)

These quotations, which are rather poignant in their own right, provide a glimpse of why two people in two cultures can be equally happy with very different quantities of goods: it is because people's utility depends not so much on what they have, as on what they have relative to the social norm.

Suppose that one accepts the notion that people care about how they compare with others, as well as what they themselves have irrespective of others (i.e., Equation 2.8). It could still be argued that, even if concern about relative position does exist, it is irrational or a character flaw that should not be respected by the analyst or policymaker. But this argument does not hold up for two reasons. First, the traditional economic theory does not evaluate where preferences come from or whether they are good or bad. Instead, it views them as what has to be satisfied in order for an individual, and ultimately a society, to be in a best-off position. Although this notion will be disputed in Section 3.2, economic theory does not view any individually held preferences pejoratively—and that would include the likes of envy, rank, or status.[14]

---

14. This tenet of modern theory also has its detractors. Joan Robinson (1962), for example, notes that under this theory, "Preference is just what the individual under discussion prefers; there is no value judgment involved. Yet, as the argument goes on, it is clear that it is a Good Thing for the individual to have what he prefers. This, it may be held, is not a question of satisfaction, but

Second, it is not at all obvious that concern about one's status compared to others is an irrational or even undesirable character trait. Tibor Scitovsky (1976) makes a strong argument to the contrary:

> The desire to "live up to the Joneses" is often criticized and its rationality called into question. This is absurd and unfortunate. Status seeking, the wish to belong, the asserting and cementing of one's membership in the group is a deep-seated and very natural drive whose origin and universality go beyond man and are explained by that most basic of drives, the desire to survive. (p. 115)

In this regard, what others have can also be viewed as necessary information for a person in formulating his or her individual desires. It shows what can be had, what is reasonable to expect.

Let us now return to the issue of how this negative externality—concern about status and rank—affects the competitive model. Recall that the advantage of competition is that it leads to Pareto optimality, where it is impossible to make someone better off without making someone else worse off. In the absence of the human characteristics being discussed here, it is easy to see the appeal of relying on competition. Why not let people engage in trade until they are satisfied with their lot and no longer wish to engage in further trades? Similarly, why not enact policies that convey benefits to some people and no cost to others? Wouldn't encouraging such trade, and enacting such policies, be in everyone's best interest?

This section has tried to show that the answer to the last question is, perhaps surprisingly, *"not necessarily."* This is because, if people feel worse off when they find themselves falling *relative* to others, then competition is not necessarily the best means of improving societal welfare. If, for example, by buying a fancy car, you make me unhappy because my car no longer seems as appealing, then society's marginal utility from your purchase of the car will be lower than your personal marginal utility. Without some sort of intervention (or intensive psychological therapy to get me to stop caring about what you have), a competitive market will overproduce goods and services that convey status.

Normally, when an externality exists, economists try to come up with taxes or subsidies that can correct it. In this case, however, there is

---

freedom—we want him to have what he prefers so as to avoid having to restrain his behaviour. But drug-fiends should be cured; children should go to school. How do we decide what preferences should be respected and what restrained unless we judge the preferences themselves? It is quite impossible for us to do that violence to our own natures to refrain from value judgments" (p. 49). This echoes the sentiments of Pigou (1932), who wrote, "Of different acts of consumption that yield equal satisfaction, one may exercise a debasing, and another an elevating influence" (p. 17).

little that can be done. One could, in theory, enact taxes on all sorts of consumer goods from which people derive status and try to distribute the revenues to those who choose not to purchase them. This, however, is not only administratively infeasible, but a political impossibility.[15]

Where does all this leave us? It is my hope that the reader now has some appreciation for the notion that an economic system based on competition, and that encourages production but not necessarily the redistribution of more and more wealth, does not always make society better off. How this applies to the field of health will be covered in Section 2.3. First, however, we consider two more key assumptions in the competitive model, beginning with the one concerning positive consumption externalities. As will become clear, those arguments will bear close resemblance to the ones just made.

2.2.2 Positive Externality: Concern about Others

In this section we deal with a different type of consumption externality: *concern about the well-being of others*. If we care about other people's needs as well as our own—be they specific ones like food or medical care, or somewhat more vague concerns about how happy the people are—then there is a positive externality of consumption. As noted earlier, a competitive market, by itself, will not provide enough of the goods and services for which there is a positive externality.

The previous section argued that people are concerned about their status relative to others. But even if we accept this, there is no reason to believe that they cannot also be concerned about others' well-being at the same time. It is perfectly natural to expect that people might have both a concern that others should have certain things like adequate food or medical care or even happiness, and also a sense of envy when others have things that they themselves do not possess. Most plausible, perhaps, would be that people want those who have less than they have to have more—although not as much as themselves, as evidenced by the Mencken quotation—and, at the same time, want to have as much as those who have more.

It is important to understand that, even though we are talking about concern for others, our focus here is also on issues of *economic efficiency*. We noted earlier that a competitive market is not designed to improve the

---

15. In that regard, Frank (1985) suggests that consumption taxes be levied on those goods that have a strong status appeal. He writes, "When relative standing is important, taxing the goods people buy serves to *remove* a distortion from economic life, not create one" (p. 249). But he does not propose how the revenue could be redistributed to those who are negatively affected by others' status goods. Even more problematic is the fact that status can be derived by innumerable commodities, not just through luxury goods.

distribution of resources among the population, so one might ask how its failure to deal with distributional issues can be raised as an efficiency problem.

The answer to this question is that there are, in actuality, two distinct reasons for redistributing income.[16] The one that might be most familiar to readers concerns issues of *social* or *distributive justice*—in essence, that redistribution is the "right thing to do." John Rawls's (1971) famous book, *A Theory of Justice* (discussed further in Chapter 5), provides a strong philosophical foundation for such a belief.

The economic tools provided earlier help illustrate the concept of social justice. Refer back to the Edgeworth Box in Figure 2.7. Suppose we are at economically efficient point *C*, where Jane has most of the wealth and Paul has little. If one views this situation, for some reason, as unfair, a possible justification for redistributing income from Jane to Paul would be to correct this inequity. Much of Chapter 5 will be devoted to examining these issues.

There is, however, a second possible reason for redistributing resources: to improve economic efficiency. Suppose that I care about poor people and want them to have more food and medical care. In order to increase my own utility, I would want to give some of my resources to the poor, stopping at the point that the marginal utility that I gain from contributing the last dollar equals the marginal utility I attain from spending it on something else.

The obvious question that arises is, why doesn't everyone just donate their optimal amount to charity, which in turn should maximize their personal utility? The problem is that many if not most people will attempt to become "free riders," which in turn will result in less redistribution than is optimal. Assume again that people care about others and want the poor to have more food, housing, medical care, and so forth. If this is done through a competitive model, an unfortunate thing happens. The Joneses will recognize that the poor will do about as well if everyone except the Joneses provides donations. But if many or most people act in this way, too little money is redistributed. The outcome therefore remains inefficient; society would be better off if there were a way to redistribute the optimal amount of resources rather than the lesser amount that occurs under competition.

There is a standard "answer" to this problem in traditional economics. That is to rely on a competitive marketplace to allocate resources efficiently, and then to employ just the right amount of special kinds of taxes

---

16. A good discussion of the distinction can be found in Wagstaff and van Doorslaer (1992).

and subsidies to redistribute income. These are called *lump-sum* taxes and subsidies.

It is important to understand the nature of these lump-sum transfers. The idea is to come up with a way to tax, say, the wealthy, to subsidize, perhaps, the poor, without changing in any important way the efficiency-enhancing incentives of a competitive market. If no such methods are feasible, then use of market competition becomes problematic when there are consumption externalities: if we do not redistribute income, the market is inefficient because people want poorer people to be better off than they are. But if we do redistribute income, we damage the efficiency that the marketplace is designed to create.

The problem with this "lump-sum solution" is the virtual impossibility of establishing true lump-sum taxes and subsidies. The idea is to come up with a way of transferring income that does not affect the incentives of either the payor of the tax, or the recipient of the subsidy.[17]

Dealing first with alternative taxation schemes, the taxes that we use most commonly do not meet this requirement because they will alter incentives. An income tax, for example, results in a reduction in net wages from the provision of additional labor. In standard theory, laborers are assumed to work until their *opportunity cost*—forgone leisure—equals the wage rate. If net wages go down from the imposition of an income tax, workers are likely to substitute more leisure for labor because the cost of labor will be lower. This results in a lower overall production of goods and services. The other common tax employed is a sales tax. The problem with a sales tax is that it results in the consumer paying a higher price than will be received by the producer. But a condition of Pareto optimality was that consumers' marginal rates of substitution must be equal to the economy's marginal rate of transformation. This is no longer the case when there is a sales tax; allowing competition to take place with sales taxes in place will not result in an economically efficient allocation of resources (Nath 1969).

Regarding the receipt of subsidies, it is equally difficult to come up with an incentive-neutral method. If we want to transfer money to the poor, a typical way of doing so is through welfare payments. But providing welfare payments to the poor results in a work disincentive. If you get a smaller welfare check when your income rises, this is no different than facing an income tax; as we just saw, a competitive market with income taxes is not economically efficient. (This, it turns out, is one of the reasons

---

17. For further discussion on problems in enacting such taxes and subsidies, see: Graaff (1971, 77–82); and Samuelson (1947, 247–49).

that we will argue for the superiority of in-kind over in-cash transfers for the poor, in Chapter 5.)

There is, in theory, one sort of tax and subsidy that might work, but it has no practicality. This is a *poll tax*—a tax that is levied irrespective of income. But as Graaff (1971) writes, a poll tax

> is not very helpful in securing desired redistributions unless we tax different men differently. But on what criteria should we discriminate between different men? Ethical ones? And what if a man cannot pay the tax? If we start taxing the poor less than the rich, we are simply reintroducing an income-tax. If we tax able men more than dunderheads, we open the door to all forms of falsification: we make stupidity seem profitable—and any able man can make himself seem stupid. Unless we really do have an omniscient observing economist to judge men's capabilities, or a slave-market where the prices they fetch reflect expert appraisals of their capacities, any taxing authority is bound to be guided by elementary visible criteria like age, marital status and—above all—ability to pay. We are back with an income tax. (p. 78)

The problem gets even more ticklish when we consider issues of fairness. Suppose we decide to tax people based not on their income, per se, but rather on their *ability* to generate income. This would mean that those who are least able to earn would be taxed less than those more able. As Paul Samuelson (1947) notes,

> Analytically, the problem resembles that of determining . . . a fair "handicap" for golfers of different ability. We wish to equalize opportunity for all contestants, but we do not want them to hold back from playing their best because of a fear of losing their favorable handicap. . . . Thus, we might decide that everyone should have at least a minimum income, that Society will make up the deficiency between what the less fortunate can earn and this minimum. Once this is realized by those who fall below the minimum, there is no longer an incentive for them to work at the margin, at least in pecuniary material terms. This is clearly bad social policy. . . . (pp. 247–48)

The foregoing discussion has been aimed at showing the near impossibility of devising workable lump-sum taxes and subsidies—which are necessary if we are to retain economic efficiency in the wake of externalities of consumption. What, then, are the implications of this dilemma? Simply this: in making policy, it is impossible to separate issues of resource allocation from issues of resource distribution. Rather, they both must be dealt with simultaneously.[18] Thurow (1980) states this nicely:

---

18. This is one of the key points of Rawls's (1971) book, *A Theory of Justice*. He argues that we must start with an allocation of "primary goods" that is based on principles of fairness. Once that is achieved, it is not inappropriate to use the market mechanism to achieve an efficient allocation of resources. Section 5.2 discusses these issues in more detail.

Decisions about economic equity are the fundamental starting point for any market economy. Individual preferences determine market demands for goods and services, but these individual preferences are weighted by incomes before being communicated to the market. An individual with no income or wealth may have needs and desires, but he has no economic resources. To make his or her personal preferences felt, he must have these resources. If income and wealth are distributed in accordance with equity (whatever that may be), individual preferences are properly weighed, and the market can efficiently adjust to an equitable set of demands. If income and wealth are not distributed in accordance with equity, individual preferences are not properly weighted. The market efficiently adjusts, but to an inequitable set of demands. . . . One way or the other, we are forced to reveal our collective preferences about what constitutes a just distribution of economic resources. (pp. 194–95)

This anomaly—the impossibility of separating allocative and distributional activities of the economy—has been raised in a variety of contexts by several economists, but has received little attention from the profession at large.[19] But if this is the case, then the traditional economic method, in which competitive forces are allowed to prevail and distribution is only done afterward, is not necessarily appropriate—especially in the presence of consumption externalities.

An example will help clarify why this is so. Suppose that a market economy reaches a Pareto-optimal state, but that this does not result in society's ideal distribution of income. (We might, for example, be at point C in Figure 2.7 but prefer to be at point B.) Consequently, it is necessary to employ taxes to redistribute income, but recall from the above discussion that there are no feasible lump-sum taxes. Instead, we use the conventional method—an income tax.

But if we use an income tax (or, for that matter, any feasible tax) to redistribute income, we saw earlier that the economy would no longer be in an optimally efficient state. If the allocation of resources was efficient before the redistribution, it would no longer be afterward. But without

---

19. Arrow (1963b), for example, has stated that, "If . . . the actual market differs significantly from the competitive model, or if the assumptions of the two optimality theorems are not fulfilled, the separation of allocative and distributional procedures becomes, in most cases, impossible" (p. 942). The two optimality conditions referred to by Arrow are that (if certain assumptions are met): (1) a competitive equilibrium is Pareto optimal; and (2) any Pareto optimum can be reached by a competitive equilibrium corresponding to a particular initial distribution of resources.

Similarly, Mishan (1969b) writes, "Far from an optimum allocation of resources representing some kind of an ideal output separable from and independent of interpersonal comparisons of welfare, a particular output retains its optimum characteristics only insofar as we commit ourselves to the particular welfare distribution uniquely associated with it" (p. 133).

Finally, Blackorby and Donaldson (1990) note that separating allocative and distributive decisions "require[s] a notion of efficiency that is independent of the distribution of income—an idea that makes no sense in real-world economies" (p. 490).

carrying out the redistribution, society would still have a suboptimal income distribution—which would mean that social welfare would be lower than it could be.

This concern would be eased if income were redistributed to the degree desired by members of society. But if it is not, then other strategies are necessary to deal with both the inefficiencies and inequities that arise when there are positive externalities of consumption. One of the best ways to deal with Thurow's concern is to enact policies that ensure that those in need obtain goods and services even if they do not have the economic resources to purchase them in the marketplace. Programs like Medicare and Medicaid—which are not in keeping with some economists' recommendations to rely on competition and then redistribute resources through cash subsidies—offer good examples of how society grapples with problems like these. More health implications are provided in Section 2.3.

2.2.3 Consumer Tastes are Predetermined

Of all of the assumptions in the traditional economic model, perhaps the one that is most often forgotten is the notion that consumers' tastes are already established when they enter the marketplace. It turns out that this assumption is extraordinarily important. This section will attempt to show that ignoring established taste is not realistic, and that when it is dropped, the competitive model loses many of its advantages.

Economics is almost universally viewed as a social science. The common element among all social sciences is that they seek to understand how individuals and/or groups of people behave. But each has its own way of viewing human behavior. Sociology, for example, focuses on how behavior is affected by society's organization, social stratification, group dynamics, and the like (Mechanic 1979). Political science examines how individuals and groups attempt to obtain what they want through such means as "conflict, influence, and authoritative collective decision making in both public and private settings" (Marmor and Dunham 1983, 3). Social psychology attempts to understand "the influences that people have upon the beliefs or behavior of others" (Aronson 1972, 6).

One facet of these other social sciences is that, in general, they seek to determine how people and groups *actually* behave. In contrast, Thurow (1983) contends, "while the reverse is true in the other social sciences that study real human behavior, prescription dominates description in economics" (p. 216). In this regard, in economics one commonly sees the word "ought" (e.g., people ought to maximize their utility, or otherwise they are being "irrational;" to maximize social welfare a society "ought" to depend on a competitive marketplace).

According to Gary Becker (1979), three things distinguish economics from the other social sciences. First, economics assumes that people engage in "maximizing behavior"; that is, individuals strive to obtain the most utility possible, firms work for the greatest profits, and so on. Second, the milieu in which people operate is the market. And third, according to Becker, is that "preferences are assumed not to change substantially over time, nor to be very different between wealthy and poor persons, or even between persons in different societies and cultures" (p. 9).[20] Similarly, Stigler and Becker (1977) go even farther than this, claiming that

> tastes neither change capriciously nor differ importantly between people. . . . [O]ne does not argue over tastes for the same reason that one does not argue over the Rocky Mountains—both are there, will be there next year, too, and are the same for all men. (p. 76)[21]

Not only are preferences assumed to be immutable, but they are also assumed to be predetermined, that is, determined outside of the economic or even social system in which the person exists. In economic theory, individual tastes and preferences "simply exist—fully developed and immutable" (Thurow 1983, 219). This is what Kenneth Boulding (1969) has referred to as the "Immaculate Conception of the Indifference Curve," because "tastes are simply given, and . . . we cannot inquire into the process by which they are formed" (p. 2).

Milton Friedman (1962) provides one explanation for this, which is consistent with the previous discussion of how economics differs from the other social sciences:

> [E]conomic theory proceeds largely to take wants as fixed . . . primarily [as] a case of division of labor. The economist has little to say about the formation of wants; this is the province of the psychologist. *The economist's task is to trace the consequences of any given set of wants.* (p. 13, italics added)[22]

Henry Aaron (1994) has pointed out one of the problems with this viewpoint, when individuals' behavior influences, and is influenced by, the community. He notes that

---

20. This point is further explored in Section 3.2.2.

21. Stigler and Becker (1977) imply that there is no need for social scientists other than economists. Recall that demand is a function of prices, incomes, and tastes. If tastes do not differ between people or change over time, all consumer behavior can be determined simply by understanding changes in price and income. Indeed, they argue that "the economist continues to search for differences in prices or incomes to explain any differences or changes in behavior" (p. 76).

22. Becker (1979) provides a second explanation for this assumption: "The assumption of stable preferences provides a stable foundation for generating predictions about responses to various changes, and prevents the analyst from succumbing to the temptation of simply postulating the required shift in preferences to 'explain' all apparent contradictions to his predictions" (p. 9).

It is then essential to recognize how changes in individual beliefs and values alter the environment in which individual actions occur. The environment is important both because people's preferences are shaped by pressure from peers and neighbors and because community attitudes shape the actual pay-offs to various kinds of individual behavior. (p. 7)

It is beyond the scope of this book to fully demonstrate that people's tastes and behaviors are mutable. Indeed, the field of social psychology is devoted, to a large extent, to this particular issue. Good overviews of the field, as well as evidence from some of the more noteworthy experiments, are provided in Aronson (1972) and Ross and Nisbett (1991).

There is overwhelming evidence that people's decisions—market-related ones and otherwise—can indeed be influenced by their environment. Consider the case of advertising. The reader, who is likely well versed in the tactics of the media, probably will admit that most consumer advertising is not aimed at providing objective information for the purposes of minimizing consumers' search for the best value. Rather, it is designed to (1) *minimize* the search process itself, and more generally, (2) change consumer tastes, in part by exerting social pressure. It is hard to claim that the tastes people come to have, as the result of exposure to this sort of advertising, are sacrosanct. In fact, people often make "bad" or nonmaximizing decisions by acting on the message—the hallmark of a successful advertising campaign!

Although it does not deal with market behavior directly, one particular set of social psychology experiments are reviewed here because they show, so graphically, how people's beliefs and behaviors can be so distorted by their environment. These are Stanley Milgram's (1963) famous studies of obedience in the face of authority.[23] These results have been used to explain, among other things, the behavior of Nazi officials during the Holocaust (Ross and Nisbett 1991).

In one version of the experiment (Milgram 1963), 40 male volunteers ages 20 to 50 are solicited to participate in a study of memory and learning at Yale University. An "experimenter" has two other individuals—one a naïve subject and the other an imposter—draw lots to determine who will be the "teacher" and the other the "learner." By design, the naïve subject always becomes the teacher, and is instructed to give electrical shocks to the learner (who is stationed in a different room) when the latter provides incorrect answers on a memory test. Although the shocks are, of course, fake, participants apparently believe that they are real, being told that

---

23. According to Lee Ross (1988), "Perhaps more than any other empirical contributions to the history of social science, [Milgram's] have become part of our society's shared intellectual legacy— that small body of historical incidents, biblical parables, and classic literature that serious thinkers feel free to draw on when they debate about human nature or contemplate human history" (p. 101).

"although the shocks can be extremely painful, they cause no permanent tissue damage" (Milgram 1963, 373). The experimenter tells the teacher to administer a shock of 15 volts for the first wrong answer, and to increase this by 15 volts each time a subsequent wrong answer is given, up to a maximum of 450 volts. The apparatus that supposedly gives the shocks has been labeled to indicate their severity, going from as low as "slight shock" to as high as "danger: severe shock." At a purported shock of 300 volts, the victim starts banging on the walls, begging that the experiment be discontinued. After 315 volts, even these protests stop, at which point the victim no longer provides any answers. But the subjects are urged by the experimenter to continue because no answer is to be construed as a wrong answer, until the maximum 450 volts is administered.

Not surprisingly, as the experiment proceeds, some subjects question the experimenter about whether they should go on, and/or whether the recipient of the shocks is all right. When this occurs, the instructor insists that they continue to participate, although no loud voice or threats are used.[24]

Much to the surprise of the researchers (and subsequently, to most of the civilized world as well), most people continued to administer shocks all the way to the maximum level. In the study referred to here, all 40 participants continued to shock the victim up to a level of 300 volts, and 35 continued even after the wall banging. A full 26 (65 percent) continued to the maximum 450 volts.

It is especially curious that subjects continued to administer the shocks given that they were clearly not predisposed to such behavior. As Milgram (1963) reports,

> Many subjects showed signs of nervousness in the experimental situation, and especially upon administering the more powerful shocks. In a large number of cases the degree of tension reached extremes that are rarely seen in sociopsychological laboratory studies. Subjects were observed to sweat, tremble, stutter, bit their lips, groan, and dig their fingernails into their flesh. . . . One sign of tension was the regular occurrence of nervous laughing fits. . . . The laughter seemed entirely out of place, even bizarre. . . . In the post-experimental interviews subjects took pains to point out that they were not sadistic types, and that the laughter did not mean they enjoyed shocking the victim. (p. 375)

Why people can be influenced to behave in a way that so contradicts their personal values has been debated for years and has still not been satisfactorily explained (Ross 1988). (Milgram himself offered 13 reasons

---

24. When questioned, the experimenter would say "please continue." If the subject balked, he would then say, in order, "the experiment requires that you continue," "it is absolutely essential that you continue," and "you have no other choise, you *must* go on" (Milgram 1963, 374).

in his 1963 article.) Some of the reasons clearly reflect the peculiar nature of the situation in which subjects found themselves.[25] The point being made here is that people's behaviors are not predetermined or fixed, but rather are subject to innumerable cognitive and social forces.

Why, then, does economics consider tastes predetermined and fixed rather than subject to the forces of change? Readers who are most familiar with economic theory will understand one possible reason. The primary tenet of modern economics is the sanctity of consumer choice. Most economists believe that the consumer is the best judge of what will maximize his or her utility. Consequently, to maximize overall social welfare, we should set up an economic system that is best at allowing consumer choices to be satisfied. Where these choices come from, as Friedman said, is beside the point.

But if what you want depends on what you had in the past, or on the influence of peers or advertisers, then it is not clear that a competitive marketplace is the best way to make people better off (Pollak 1978). It is true that, if certain conditions are met, a competitive market will result in allocative efficiency. However, there is a major caveat attached to this—that the things people demand are really the ones that will make them best off. We pursue this issue more broadly in Chapter 3. Here, we focus on the specific issue of whether satisfying consumers' tastes, as indicated by their demand for particular goods and services, will necessarily maximize their utility.

In the paragraphs below, three examples are provided in which people's market behaviors are not predetermined but rather are a result of their past or present environments. In each case, it is not clear that fulfillment of their personal choices would make them best off.

The first example, and perhaps the least important of the three given, concerns addiction. Suppose that, while growing up, you are in a peer group that smokes cigarettes and you become addicted. Once you leave that peer group, you will still have a "taste" for cigarettes and are more likely to demand them than someone who is not addicted. Can we really say, in such an instance, that satisfying this "taste" through the marketplace is efficient from a societal standpoint—in the same way as satisfying the demand for bread or literature? Might not you be better

---

25. The experiment was sponsored by a noted university; it was purportedly for a worthy purpose—to study how to enhance learning; the "victim" supposedly volunteered and was randomly chosen to be the recipient of the shocks; the experimenter did not bend in his conviction that the subject continue administering the shocks; the subject is told that no permanent physical damage will result from the shocks, etc. (Milgram 1963).

off if cigarettes were taxed so prohibitively (or even banned) that you stopped smoking?[26]

A second and much more general application is habit formed by past consumption patterns.[27] Suppose you live in a community that has not discovered the joys of music. A resident of such a place will therefore not have developed a taste for music. But, as Alfred Marshall (1920), another of the fathers of modern economics, once noted, "the more good music a man hears, the stronger is his taste for it likely to become" (p. 94). The aforementioned resident might likely be better off with music than without, but he or she has not been sufficiently "educated" to know this.[28,29]

This is a very big problem for competitive markets. If people demand goods based on their prior experience—as they certainly must—and furthermore, if their prior experience is colored by the economic environment in which they live, then they will demand the things that tend to be characteristic of that environment. That implies a strong advantage for whatever is the status quo; familiarity breeds preference (as opposed to breeding contempt), so what exists now will be demanded in the future.

If one believes that tastes are determined in such a way, then it becomes clear that a society might be better off pursuing some goods and services that are not demanded most strongly by the public. This is because people might not know what alternatives are available that will make them better off, but to which they have not be exposed in the past. But if consumer tastes are viewed as predetermined, as they are in the economic model, people become "stuck" with whatever they demand because they are assumed always to know best.

The third example concerns occupational choices. In the traditional economic model, it is assumed that people make occupational choices based on weighing all alternatives; factors considered would include how much satisfaction they obtain from the work and the wages that it offers. Whatever choice is made in a competitive labor market is assumed to be

---

26. Note that this argument does not hinge on the negative externalities associated with smoking. Prohibitive taxes could also be enacted so that there are fewer negative side effects on others as a result of your smoking.

27. For a good discussion of these issues, see Hahnel and Albert (1990).

28. Stated in economic terms, the tangency between their indifference curve and budget constraint is not utility maximizing.

29. The idea of having the economic system not only reflect given preferences, but also nurture "more refined" preferences, has been a theme of some radical economists. Herbert Gintis (1970), for example, has said that a person can use his existing preferences to demand what he has demanded before, or alternatively, "*improve* his preference structure so as to be capable of increased satisfaction based on available material goods" (p. 12). Gintis believes that the commodities that are contained in people's utility functions should not be viewed as ends in themselves, but rather, instruments for obtaining higher welfare; he attacks conventional welfare economists as "commodity fetishists."

utility maximizing. But this might not be the case if tastes are a product of one's environment.

Suppose, for example, that a person grows up in a factory town and later decides to work in the factory. This might not necessarily be utility maximizing; it is possibly a poor choice, made because of the person's limited horizons. As another example, imagine that one person works to perform house-cleaning services for another. This may not reflect the personal preferences of the worker as much as lack of good alternatives (Buchanan 1977). In this regard, John Roemer (1994) states that "people learn to live with what they are accustomed to or what is available to them. . . . Thus the slave may have adapted to like slavery; welfare judgments based on individual preferences are clearly impugned in such situations" (p. 120). The status quo would be favored by competitive markets, even though people might be better off if society, in some way, intervened in these choices. (A public job-training program would be an example.)

In summary, this discussion has tried to show that encouraging consumer choice through competitive markets might not always be the best way of raising people's and society's welfare, if people have strong positive or negative feelings about the possessions of others, or if their tastes are malleable rather than predetermined. The next section considers some examples of how these assumptions affect health policy.

2.3 Implications for Health Policy

This chapter has attempted to show that economic theory does not provide a strong justification for the superiority of competitive policies in the health area. This is because the competitive model is based on certain important assumptions that, we argued, do not appear to be met. This section provides some implications of these conclusions for health policy.

2.3.1 Equalizing Access to Health Services

Market forces operate through individuals' desires to gain from trade. If someone wishes to enter the marketplace to engage in such trading, economic theory shows that allowing that person to do so will increase his or her welfare without reducing that of others—which, in turn, will make society better off. This is true, however, only if there are no significant negative consumption externalities associated with the person's consumption.

At first glance, it might appear that most developed countries embrace this individualistic viewpoint when it comes to health policy.

Practically all countries, even those with comprehensive universal health insurance programs, allow their citizens to spend their own money on additional health services if those citizens wish to go outside of the government-sanctioned program. But on closer examination, it can be demonstrated that health policy has been conducted on quite contrary principles. This is true even in the United States, where, it will be argued, society has, up until now, tried to minimize large differences in access to care. One concern, however, is whether future U.S. health policy will embrace the competitive ethic too literally. As noted in Chapter 1, the rate of uninsurance among the nonelderly population is on the rise (Employee Benefits Research Institute 1996), in part because of competitive pressures on providers and insurers. This leads to a situation in which more people without insurance see themselves as disadvantaged in comparison with others. The concern here is that a continuation of this trend will result in even more of the negative externalities that previous policy has tried to reduce.

Evidence supporting the viewpoint that U.S. health policy has eschewed the competitive prescription dates back many years. Beginning with the post–World War II period, the subsidization of the building and expansion of hospitals under the Hill-Burton Act (1948), and subsequent subsidization of physician training costs, directly reflected a belief that poorer, rural areas of the United States should not be disadvantaged *relative to* wealthier, urban areas of the country. By defining the need for hospitals based on the per capita availability of beds, the philosophy behind Hill-Burton was that no areas of the country should be given greater access than others to hospital care.[30]

More recent evidence is provided by state mandates concerning the content of health insurance coverage. An implication of the competitive model is that insurance companies are allowed to provide whatever health insurance coverage they wish. In fact, this is not the case; states, which have almost all regulatory authority over the sale of insurance, have enacted numerous "mandates" concerning the eligibility for, and content of, health insurance policies. One study found that by 1988, there were more than 730 mandates across the different states (Gabel and Jensen 1989). It reported, for example, that 37 states require insurers to cover alcohol treatment, 28 require that mental health services be covered, and 18, maternity care. It is true that special interest groups provide much

---

30. In fact, because of greater driving distances in rural areas, subsidies were aimed at giving them higher bed-to-population ratios than urban areas. The construction and expansion of hospitals was subsidized up to a level of 5.5 beds per 1,000 people in areas where there were fewer than 6 persons per square mile, versus only 4.5 beds per 1,000 in areas exceeding 12 persons per square mile.

of the support for these mandates; nevertheless, consumer groups, and particularly people who need certain services (or know someone who does), also tend to support them.

Similar evidence can be seen by examining the political fallout that arose from the Oregon proposal for Medicaid reform, which was dubbed as requiring "rationing" of services. Early versions of the proposal engendered a great deal of opposition, mainly because program beneficiaries would not be able to receive coverage for the same services as the rest of the population. Rather, what services would be paid for would depend on how much money was available. Less cost-effective services would not be covered if program money was exhausted after paying for more cost-effective services. This prompted Bruce Vladeck (1990), who later became director of the federal government's Health Care Financing Administration, to write,

> [T]his will be the first system in memory to explicitly plan that poor people with treatable illnesses will die if Medicaid runs out of money or does not budget correctly, and providers will be excused from liability for failing to treat them. The Oregonians argue that it is healthier for society to make such choices explicitly, but it is hardly healthy to establish rules of the game that require such choices. (p. 3)

In fact, the proposal was cleared by federal officials only after the methodology was revised to ensure that disabled individuals would not face discrimination in coverage (Fox and Leichter 1993), and after the state made it clear that all essential services would be provided.[31]

A final example of how U.S. health policy operates in conflict with the competitive model concerns coverage for new technologies. Imagine that a new technology becomes available that can help save lives, but is very expensive. Is society better off if we allow only the very rich to purchase it, as the Pareto principle would imply? It might seem that the answer is "yes," because we do allow people to spend their own money for such procedures so long as the procedures are not illegal. But on further reflection, it becomes clear that something quite different is going on.

Traditionally, when new and potentially effective technologies become available, they are viewed as experimental until their safety and efficacy are established. But once established, insurers almost always cover them; failure to do so results first in strong pressure from policyholders, and eventually in lawsuits that the insurer is withholding necessary medical care. Having these technologies covered by public and

---

31. Politics undoubtedly entered the decision as well. The Bush administration had blocked approval of the plan, but soon after taking office, the Clinton administration approved it. See Pollak et al. (1994).

private insurance ensures that access to them is available to the large majority of the population that has health insurance. In this regard, Uwe Reinhardt (1992) writes,

> Suppose [that a] new, high-tech medical intervention [is available] and that more of it could be produced without causing reductions in the output of any other commodity. Suppose next, however, that the associated rearrangement of the economy has been such that only well-to-do patients will have access to the new medical procedure. On these assumptions, can we be sure that [this] would enhance overall *social welfare*? Would we not have to assume the absence of *social envy* among the poor and of guilt among the well-to-do? Are these reasonable assumptions? Or should civilized policy analysts refuse to pay heed to base human motives such as envy, prevalent though it may be in any normal society? (p. 311)

If public policy were based on market competition, then we would see a gap between the services that are available to the wealthy and those available to the rest of the insured population. We do not see such a gap; once a procedure is found to be safe and effective, everyone with private health insurance is potentially eligible to receive it. And, if insurers are not sufficiently quick to adopt new procedures, states can and do mandate their provision.[32]

This is not to say that policy has ensured equal access for all Americans. In fact, the uninsured population tends to use few services and to benefit from fewer new medical technologies than others (Wenneker, Weismann, and Epstein 1990; Braveman et al. 1991). Up until now, however, most have been able to benefit from a safety net of public hospitals and community clinics, as well as "cross-subsidization" of uninsured patients by their insured counterparts.

One consequence of the increasingly competitive medical marketplace in the United States is a breakdown in the public health system, coupled with reduced cross-subsidization of the uninsured. To keep costs down, private hospitals are sending more of their sickest indigent patients to public hospitals, which in turn find themselves in increasing financial distress (Thorpe 1997). Private insurers (spurred in part by employers, who foot much of the bill) are less willing to pay providers enough to allow them to care for those without coverage. Thus, although U.S. public policy has tried in the past to keep differences in access to care from becoming large, increased competition in the health sector appears to

---

32. States cannot currently mandate provision of services under employer-sponsored health plans that fall under the jurisdiction of the Employee Retirement Income and Security Act (ERISA). Although this has effectively reduced the strength of state mandates, there is little doubt that such mandates would still exist if ERISA were repealed.

be working in the opposite direction—which, we have argued, is not consistent with raising social welfare in the presence of externalities of consumption.

2.3.2 What Comes First: Allocation or Distribution?

As noted above, in the traditional economic paradigm, a competitive market is used to ensure that resources are allocated efficiently. But if there are positive externalities of consumption—for example, if society wants poorer people to have more resources—then the free-rider effect will prevent a competitive economy from achieving allocative efficiency. The solution to this problem under the economic model is to institute lump-sum taxes and subsidies, because they do not distort incentives and reduce efficiency; but in practice, no such mechanisms are available.

A more reasonable approach to dealing with this problem is for society to grapple with allocative and distributive issues concurrently. Rather than saying, "we will take whatever the competitive market gives us, and then institute the necessary taxes and subsidies," a reasonable society might contend that "we will start with certain redistributive principles, and once they are established, allow the market to operate around these principles."

Reinhardt (1992) provides a similar philosophy:

> [T]o begin an exploration of alternative proposals for the reform of our health system without first setting forth explicitly, and very clearly, the *social values* to which the reformed system is to adhere strikes at least this author as patently *inefficient*: it is a waste of time. Would it not be more *efficient* merely to explore the *relative efficiency* of alternative proposals that do conform to widely shared *social values*? (p. 315)

This method—rather than the method advocated through the competitive model—is how policy has traditionally been made in the United States as well as almost all developed countries. In the United States, public programs like Medicare and Medicaid were established *outside* of the competitive marketplace in order to ensure that our priority—access to medical care services for the elderly and the poor—was met.

The belief that we should start with principles of fairness, and then proceed to considerations of efficiency, is also the foundation on which most other health systems have been built. In their comprehensive study of financing and equity in nine health systems in Europe and the United States, Adam Wagstaff and Eddy van Doorslaer (1992) found that:

> [t]here appears to be broad agreement . . . among policy-makers in at least eight of the nine European countries [studied] that payments towards health care should be related to ability to pay rather than to use of medical facilities.

Policy-makers in all nine European countries also appear to be committed to the notion that all citizens should have access to health care. In many countries this is taken further, it being made clear that access to and receipt of health care should depend on need, rather than on ability to pay. (p. 363)

Returning to the United States, there has been a resurgence of late in relying on health maintenance organizations (HMOs) and other competitive policies in both the Medicare and Medicaid programs. Although such policies may bring about cost savings, there is concern that their enactment will reduce access for some of the poor and elderly—which, as was argued, has up until now increased social welfare due to the positive externalities associated with coverage for these groups. This is not because they would lose coverage; rather, it stems from a concern that the two groups that may be least able to "navigate" their way through HMOs' gatekeeping systems are poor and elderly persons (Ware et al. 1986; Ware et al. 1996). The overall concern is that the reliance on more competition will jeopardize the principles that formed the basis of these programs in the first place.

2.3.3 Competition and Prevention

Another manifestation of the problems associated with the free-rider effect concerns prevention. Traditionally, HMOs have encouraged preventive services both through low service copayments, and by covering services not traditionally included in many fee-for-service health plans, such as annual preventive examinations and diagnostic tests. One of the reasons HMOs have given for providing these services to members is that such services will reduce future health-related costs. This will not be the case, however, if plan members regularly switch between competing (and often nearly identical) health plans. In this regard, Donald Light (1995) writes,

> prevention by any given [health] plan only makes economic sense within a contract year, or else one's competitors may benefit from one's efforts when subscribers switch plans in the next contract year. . . . Why should a given plan, for example, make efforts to reduce drug abuse or smoking at the schools of a given town when only some of the children are their customers, and their parents may move or switch plans next year? (p. 151)

Recent data show that individuals are willing to switch their health plans in the wake of very small premium differences—particularly when there are few discernible differences between these alternatives (Buchmueller and Feldstein 1996; Christianson et al. 1995).[33]

---

33. Individual practice associations often have very similar provider panels, so it would not be clear to most consumers that the plan they chose would make much of a difference. There may,

It is too early to know whether, in fact, the provision of preventive services is indeed declining as a result of this free-rider effect. Documentation of such an effect would provide further reason to consider limiting the number of health plan choices available to consumers, or to move toward a more publicly funded system.[34]

2.3.4 Government-Sponsored Health Education

The traditional economic model assumes that consumer tastes are predetermined. People come into the marketplace knowing what they want, and what they want is intrinsic to them; it is not shaped by past consumption or by external forces.

How does advertising fit into all of this? There are really two types of advertising: that designed to provide purely objective information (e.g., prices, availability) and that aimed at shaping consumer tastes. Advertisers may pass along information to the consumer that, if accepted, will not necessarily be in the consumer's best interest.

One policy implication of this concerns health education. Because economics concerns itself primarily with money-type variables (e.g., price, insurance, income), its practitioners tend to be less conversant about other policy interventions, such as education designed to change people's harmful habits. If, however, preferences are the product of advertisers' activities, there may be a role for medical education in undoing some of these deleterious effects.

Government has long been involved, for example, in trying to convince the public not to smoke. Part of this effort has been regulatory. Tobacco companies, for example, cannot advertise their products on television.[35] But government has also been directly involved in anti-smoking campaigns, through explicit advertisements as well as requiring tobacco companies to put various health disclosures on their packaging. One wonders if more of this, extending into other consumer behaviors (e.g., nutrition, drinking) is not warranted. The need for these efforts is heightened if consumer tastes are malleable rather than predetermined.

2.3.5 Should Cost Control be a Public Policy?

A larger issue that arises if consumer tastes are pliable concerns cost control. Health economists often point out that we cannot say that a

however, *be* substantial differences, because different plans may have different financial incentives for providers and employ different utilization monitoring techniques. For a discussion of these issues, see Hibbard, Sofaer, and Jewett (1996).

34. In this regard, Robert Kuttner (1997) writes, "A purely privatized system is likely to be more fragmented, and less willing to pay for public health, or to grasp its logic (p. 158).

35. At the time of writing, several major tobacco companies are in the midst of negotiations with states that, among other things, are designed to reduce smoking among youths and other groups.

country spends too much of its national income on health services. Who is to say that 14 percent or even 25 percent is "too much?" It is contended that nothing is necessarily wrong if a society wants to spend more of its money on, say, expensive technologies. In fact, survey data show that about half of all Americans believe that the country spends *too little* on medical care (Blendon et al. 1995b). But this viewpoint is harder to justify if one views consumer tastes not as predetermined but rather as the product of previous experiences.

Take the example of medical technology. People are likely to demand the fruits of new technologies in part because they come to expect them. Table 2.3 shows the relative availability of selected medical technologies in Canada, Germany, and the United States (Rublee 1994). For all six technologies shown, the number of units per million persons is far higher in the United States than in Canada and Germany. With regard to open-heart surgery, the figures are almost three times as high in the United States as in Canada, and nearly five times as great as in Germany. Magnetic resonance imaging, which is perhaps the most extreme example of international differences, has figures for the United States ten times as great as Canada and three times as great as Germany.

More important than the availability of technologies is whether there are differences by country in their rate of usage. Fewer data are available on this, but studies of the United States and Canada do show substantial differences. One study, which examined hospital utilization rates from eight similar hospitals in 1990, found radiology usage to be 40 percent higher in the United States, due mainly to 119 percent higher use rates for computed tomography scans and magnetic resonance imaging (Katz, McMahan, and Manning 1996). Another study that examined treatment patterns found U.S. physicians to be much more likely than Canadian physicians to recommend invasive treatments such as coronary angiography after uncomplicated myocardial infarction (Pilote et al. 1995).

Because such technologies are more available and are used more in the United States, the U.S. public is likely to have developed greater expectations of their use. Some analysts argue that it is the growth of these technologies—or, as Joseph Newhouse (1993) termed it, "the enhanced capabilities of medicine" (p. 162)—that is primarily responsible for rising health costs in the United States.

The point—that maybe people would be equally well off without so many expensive (not to say duplicative) lifesaving interventions—is made only tentatively. One would not want to claim that people want to live longer because they are inculcated into believing that is desirable. Clearly, though, quality-of-life issues become relevant to such a discussion, as

Table 2.3 Comparative Availability of Selected Medical Technologies, Canada, Germany, and United States, 1992–1993

	Canada (1993)			Germany (1993)			United States (1992)		
	Number of Units	Units per Million Persons	Change since 1989	Number of Units	Units per Million Persons	Change since 1987	Number of Units	Units per Million Persons	Change since 1987
Open-heart Surgery	36	1.3	1.3%	61	0.8	0.4%	945	3.7	2.6%
Cardiac Catheterization	78	2.8	17.0	277	3.4	4.5	1,631	6.4	4.8
Organ Transplantation	34	1.2	3.2	39	0.5	1.0	612	2.4	12.9
Radiation Therapy	132	4.8	11.0	373	4.6	6.7	2,637	10.3	2.3
Lithotripsy	13	0.5	24.0	117	1.4	27.3	480	1.9	14.9
Magnetic Resonance Imaging	30	1.1	18.6	296	3.7	25.5	2,900	11.2	20.4

Source: Rublee, D. A. 1994. "Medical Technology in Canada, Germany, and the United States: An update." *Health Affairs* 13 (4): 115.
Copyright © 1994 The People-to-People Health Foundation, Inc., All Rights Reserved.

Table 2.4 The Public's View of Their Medical Care System in Ten Nations, 1990

	Minor Changes Needed	Fundamental Changes Needed	Completely Rebuild System	Per Capita Health Expenditure (U.S. dollars)
Canada	56%	38%	5%	1,483
Netherlands	47	46	5	1,041
West Germany	41	35	13	1,093
France	41	42	10	1,105
Australia	34	43	17	939
Sweden	32	58	6	1,233
Japan	29	47	6	915
United Kingdom	27	52	17	758
Italy	12	46	40	841
United States	10	60	29	2,051

Source: Blendon, R. J. et al., 1990. "Satisfaction with Health Systems in Ten Nations." *Health Affairs* 9 (2): Ex. 2, p. 188. Copyright © 1990 The People-to-People Health Foundation, Inc. All Rights Reserved.

does the fact that the United States ranks near the top of the world in only one major vital statistic category—life expectancy after reaching age 80.[36] One must take pause when considering Easterlin's results that were presented earlier—that people in poor countries seem to be equally happy as those in wealthier ones—or perhaps more relevant to health, the fact that citizens of other countries, which spend far less money on medical care, tend to be much happier with their medical care systems. This latter point is supported by the data in Table 2.4, which shows the satisfaction that citizens in ten developed countries have in their medical care systems. Only Italians show satisfaction levels as low as Americans (Blendon et al. 1990).

This belief, that more and more spending on technologies does not seem to be increasing utility levels very much, is consistent with a rather sober quotation[37] from E. J. Mishan (1969a):

---

36. Data from 24 developed countries show that female life expectancy in the United States at age 80 is rivaled only by Canada, and male life expectancy at that age, only by Canada and Iceland. In contrast, 15 countries exceed the United States in female life expectancy at birth, and 17 in male life expectancy. See Schieber, Poullier, and Greenwald (1992).

37. Similarly, Kuttner (1997) discusses the book, *The Overworked American* by Juliet Schor, which he describes as pointing "to a vicious circle in which the pursuit of material satisfactions promised by advertising leads Americans to work more hours than they really want, in order to have money to buy the products that never quite yield their promised fulfillments. Over time, people internalize two contradictory conclusions—a cumulative cynicism combined with an unquenchable hunger that perhaps the next product will somehow yield the elusive satisfaction" (Kuttner 1997, p. 57).

As I see it, the main task today of the economist at all concerned with the course of human welfare is that of weaning the public from its post-war fixation on economic growth; of inculcating an awareness of the errors and misconceptions that abound in popular appraisals of the benefits of industrial development; and also, perhaps of voicing an occasional doubt whether the persistent pursuit of material ends, borne onwards today by a tidal wave of unrealisable expectations, can do more eventually than to agitate the current restlessness, and to add to the frustrations and disillusion of ordinary mortals. (p. 81)

DEMAND THEORY

J UST AS market competition represents the core concept in microeconomics, demand theory is the key to understanding market competition. Demand, which economists often define as how many goods and services are purchased at alternative prices, is the mechanism that drives a competitive economy. Under demand theory, the amount of a commodity that is produced and consumed is determined by people's demand for it. If people's tastes change for some reason, and they want more of one good and less of another, prices will change, prompting firms to adjust their production. Unless there is some sort of constraint on obtaining the necessary inputs for production, in the long run supply adjusts to satisfy demand.

But demand theory means more than just this. It also forms the basis by which economic theory evaluates social welfare. If people demand a certain bundle of goods and services, it means that they prefer that bundle to all other ways in which they could spend their money. In other words, the things people demand are, by definition, those things that put them at the highest level of welfare, given the resources available. And if all people act in a way that maximizes their utilities, given their available income, society will also be at a welfare maximum.[1]

Section 3.1 contains a brief summary of the traditional demand theory; readers already familiar with such concepts as social welfare, revealed preference, and consumer surplus can move on to the following

---

1. This assumes that society is satisfied with the distribution of income, which will be discussed further in this chapter as well as in Chapter 5.

section. Section 3.2 provides a critique of demand theory; this critique is based, to a large extent, on questioning the validity of some of the assumptions of demand theory that were listed in Chapter 1. Section 3.3 applies this critique to a number of health economic issues and tools that are used to draw policy conclusions about health policy.

3.1 The Traditional Economic Model

This discussion is divided into four subsections: Utility and Social Welfare; Revealed Preference; Demand Curves and Functions; and The Meaning of Demand and Consumer Surplus.

3.1.1 Utility and Social Welfare

In Section 2.1.1, we saw that under traditional economic theory, consumers are assumed to make choices about the goods and services they purchase in ways that will maximize their utility. How do we determine whether these choices will also be best for society as a whole?

Some early theorists, who collectively are known as the classical *utilitarians*, believed that total social welfare was simply the numerical sum of all individuals' welfare. The question naturally arises about how it was possible to quantify such measures. Perhaps the leading early advocate of classical utilitarianism, Jeremy Bentham (1791), thought that it was possible to measure utility through its manifestations of pleasure and pain. Of these, he wrote:

> Nature has pleased mankind under the governance of two sovereign masters, *pain* and *pleasure*. It is for them alone to point out what we ought to do, as well as to determine what we shall do. On the one hand the standard of right and wrong, on the other the chain of causes and effects, are fastened to their throne. They govern us in all we do, in all we say, in all we think: every effort we can make to throw off our subjection, will serve but to demonstrate and confirm it. (Bentham 1968, p. 3)

If everyone has the same capacity to experience pleasure and pain, and if we also assume that there is diminishing marginal utility, then an interesting policy prescription arises under classical utilitarianism: social welfare is maximized when everyone has the same income. It is easy to see why this is the case. Suppose one person has $10,000 in income and another $5,000. If an additional dollar is spent by the former person, it will bring less utility than if spent by the latter. Only if everyone has the same income will total welfare be maximized.

Although some "radical utilitarians" were comfortable with this implication, others—some of whom presumably would have lost a great deal through the equalization of incomes—were not. And it was not hard to poke holes in the theory. Classical utilitarianism is based on two important assumptions: (1) utility can be quantified, and (2) it is possible to add utilities across different individuals.

Modern economists tend to eschew both of these assumptions and have made a great deal of progress without them. (As noted in Section 5.2, economists still employ a utilitarian viewpoint, but one that makes much weaker assumptions.) The works of Pareto and Edgeworth, discussed in Section 2.1, were instrumental in this regard, as was the more recent work of Paul Samuelson. Microeconomics now proceeds under the Pareto principle, where a policy is desirable if it makes someone better off without making anyone worse off. But in order to go further—say, to advocate one program or tax over another, when there will be both winners and losers, as being better for society as a whole—explicit value judgments are necessary.

3.1.2 Revealed Preference

In Section 2.1.1, we introduced indifference curves but did not discuss where they came from. One way to derive them is to ask people which alternative bundle of goods they would prefer. But there are two problems with this technique. First, it is difficult to imagine administering such a population survey given the nearly countless possible bundles of goods from which people can choose. Second, it is entirely possible that people will not tell the truth, or even if they do, their responses may not predict their actual behavior when faced with such market choices.

The concept of *revealed preference* is designed to eliminate these problems. Under this theory, pioneered by Samuelson (1938), people are simply assumed to prefer whatever bundle of goods they choose to consume. If they purchase one bundle but could afford another one, we can say that they have revealed themselves to prefer the former. One significant aspect of this theory is that it does not rely on understanding the psyche of the individual. Rather, as Robert Sugden (1993) has noted,

> [T]he most significant property of the revealed preference approach . . . is that we do not need to enquire into the reasons why one thing is chosen rather than another. We do not look into the factors that go into the deliberation which leads to a choice; we look only at the results of that process. . . . (p. 1949)

It is possible to derive indifference curves through the theory of revealed preference; all one has to do is witness actual consumer behavior over different sets of prices and income. In doing so, economists are making an important assumption, to which we will return in Section 3.2:

whatever bundle people choose is the bundle that, at least before the fact, is expected to make them best off.

3.1.3 Demand Curves and Functions

It is not hard to go from the concept of indifference curves and revealed preference to the concept of demand. Following the example given in Chapter 2, Figure 3.1 shows three indifference curves for nurse practitioner (NP) and physician (MD) visits for a particular consumer. We then vary the price of NP visits from P_n to $P_n/2$ to $P_n/4$ but do not change the price of MD visits (P_m) or income. The result is that the budget line pivots outward. Under these three alternative sets of prices, the consumer chooses to purchase six, eight, and ten NP visits per year, respectively. These points are then plotted as a *demand curve* labeled D_1 in Figure 3.2. A demand curve shows how much of a good is purchased at alternative prices. Although one needs actual data on consumer behavior to draw such a curve accurately, in general it exhibits a downward-sloping-to-the-right shape, indicating that people will demand more when the price is lower.

We already saw that a demand curve is drawn under the assumptions that the price of other goods does not change and a person's income does

Figure 3.1 Derivation of Demand Curve, Step 1

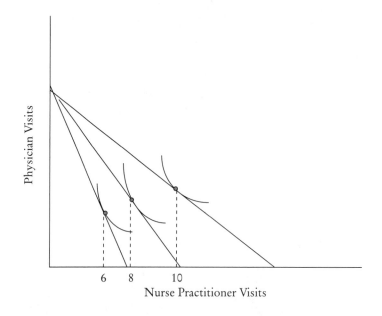

Figure 3.2 Derivation of Demand Curve, Step 2

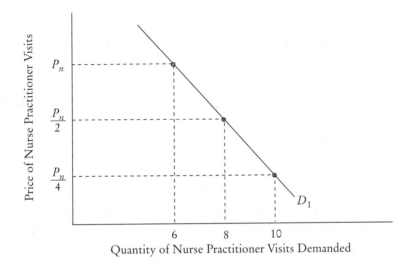

not change. It is further assumed that a person's tastes are also unaltered. In functional form:

$$D = f(P, P_a, I, T) \tag{3.1}$$

where D is demand for a particular good or service, P is its price, P_a is the price of alternatives, I is income, and T is tastes. *Aggregate* demand—how much is demanded by all individuals combined—is simply the sum of individual demands.

There are two kinds of these alternative goods: *complements* and *substitutes*. Complements are goods that are used in conjunction with the good being studied, and substitutes are ones that are used instead.[2] We can therefore refine Equation 3.1 as follows:

$$D = f(P, P^s, P^c, I, T) \tag{3.2}$$

where P^s is the price of substitutes, and P^c, the price of complements.

What is perhaps most noteworthy about these equations is the unobtrusive role played by T, tastes. Wrapped up in this variable is nearly everything that makes a person tick. Much of the research in the fields of

---

2. The technical definitions are somewhat more involved. Goods are complements if their cross-price elasticity of demand is negative; they are substitutes if it is positive. The cross-price elasticity of demand is defined as the percentage change in the quantity demanded of a particular good, divided by the percentage change in the price of another good (the complement or substitute).

psychology and sociology has been devoted to addressing how individual tastes are formed and the ways in which they are manifested. But as we noted in Section 2.2.3, economic theory takes the taste variable as predetermined and unaffected by the person's environment.

In the health area, perhaps the major component of T is health status. If people are sick, they are obviously more likely to use medical care than if they are well. In that one sense, they have more of a "taste" for health. This would not seem to be a very good way to classify your desire for medical services if, say, you are hit by a car, but there is no other place to put it if one uses Equation 3.2. As a result, sometimes one sees the demand for health written as:

$$D = f(P, P^s, P^c, I, HS, T) \tag{3.3}$$

where HS is the patient's health status. In Equation 3.3, tastes no longer capture health status, but rather only the non-health-related determinants of demand.

As we saw, a single demand curve can be used to illustrate any relationship between the quantity and price of a particular good. It is assumed, however, that the other determinants of demand—the prices of alternative goods, income, health status, and tastes—remain unchanged. If they do change, then the demand curve must also shift. For example, when a person gets sick, his or her demand curve is likely to shift outward and to the right, indicating that he or she will demand more medical care at all price levels. Nevertheless, the amount demanded is still expected to depend on the price of medical care.

The exact relationship between the quantity of a good purchased and its price is represented by the *elasticity of demand*. This is defined as the percentage change in the quantity of a good demanded, divided by the percentage change in its price. If the elasticity of demand equals −0.5, it means that when the price of the good changes by, say, 10 percent, the quantity demanded changes by 5 percent, but in the opposite direction. Much health economic research has been devoted to determining various demand elasticities for medical services.[3]

3.1.4 The Meaning of Demand and Consumer Surplus

The derivation of demand curves through indifference curves, which in turn can be derived from revealed preferences, leads to an important implication: the goods and services that people demand are the ones that, at least before the fact, are expected to make them best off. That

---

3. For a review of this evidence, see Feldstein (1988, 93–97) or Phelps (1992, ch. 5).

is to say, the act of demanding one set of goods, given prevailing prices and incomes, implies that a person is likely to be better off with that set than with any other set of goods that he or she can afford. And if this is the case, it is a fairly small leap to say then that an economic system that allows people to choose their bundles is best for society. Critiquing this proposition will be the primary purpose of Section 3.2.

It is useful, however, to try first to understand exactly what a demand curve means, which in turn will provide insights into the important concept of consumer surplus. As indicated by revealed preference, when a person demands a good, it means that he or she prefers it to all alternatives. One of these alternatives is, of course, not spending the money in the first place.

The theory therefore implies that the utility obtained from purchasing a good or service is at least as great as the price paid—or it would not have been purchased in the first place. What a demand curve therefore shows is the *marginal utility* of a particular purchase. If a person buys six apples when they are priced at 50 cents each but buys seven when they are priced at 40 cents, then the marginal utility derived from the purchase of the seventh apple is at least 40 cents.

We saw in Section 2.1.1 that consumers are assumed to try to maximize their utility through the bundle of goods that they purchase. They would therefore seek only those goods whose marginal utilities exceeded the market price. Consumers are often fortunate enough to be in a position where the market price of a good they seek is less than the maximum amount they would be willing to pay. The difference between how much consumers are willing to pay for something, and what it actually costs, is called *consumer surplus*. The concept, first used in the mid-1800s by Jules Dupuit, a French engineer, to determine the value of railroad bridges, was popularized by Alfred Marshall to the English-speaking world (Ng 1979; Parkin 1994).

The calculation of consumer surplus is illustrated in Figure 3.3. Suppose that the market price of an NP visit is $30, at which price our consumer Paul is willing to purchase four per year (point B on demand curve D_1). Note, however, that he was willing to pay much more for the first three visits: $40 for the third visit, $50 for the second, and $60 for the first. Thus, in purchasing four NP visits, Paul has earned a surplus. He was willing to pay $180 for the four visits but only had to pay $120 ($4 \times $30), so he has earned a consumer surplus of $60. This is illustrated by the triangle ABC in Figure 3.3.[4]

---

4. The size of the triangle ABC equals $80 rather than $60 because, as drawn, Paul could purchase fractions of visits as well.

Figure 3.3 Derivation of Consumer Surplus

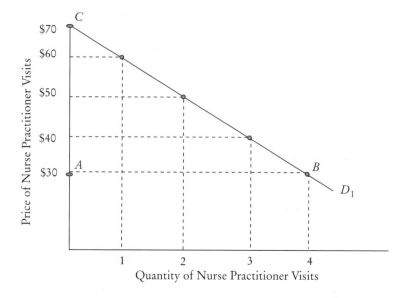

The concept of consumer surplus comes into play not so much at the individual level, but in the aggregate. If we add together all of the surpluses received by all consumers, we obtain the total consumer surplus, which is the difference between the value consumers receive from a good, and how much they have to pay for it. Economists use this tool for such matters as determining whether society should embark on a publicly financed investment or project, and in other applications such as calculating the "welfare loss" from excess health insurance, which is discussed later, in Section 3.3.1.

3.2 Problems with the Traditional Model

In *Candide*, the philosopher Dr. Pangloss attempts to prove that the obviously flawed state of nature and society is, nevertheless, the best of all possible worlds. Voltaire (1759) quotes his character as stating,

> It is demonstrated that things cannot be otherwise: for, since everything was made for a purpose, everything is necessarily for the best purpose. Note that noses were made to wear spectacles; we therefore have spectacles. Legs were clearly devised to wear breeches, and we have breeches. . . . And since pigs were made to be eaten, we have pork all year round. Therefore, those who have maintained that all is well have been talking nonsense: they should have maintained that all is for the best. (p. 18)

Although perhaps not recognized by most economists, the theory of revealed preference in particular, and consumer theory in general, bears a striking resemblance to Pangloss's philosophy.[5] By choosing a particular bundle of goods, people demonstrate that they prefer it to all others; consequently, it is best for them. And, if all people are in their best position, then society—which is simply the aggregation of all people— is also in its best position. Therefore, allowing people to choose in the marketplace results in the best of all possible economic worlds.

The purpose of this section is to demonstrate that this sort of syllogism (which will be made more explicit below) is tenuous at best because it is based on assumptions that are difficult to support, particularly in the health area. We will question the conventional meaning of the demand curve where it purports to show the marginal utility obtained by consumers through the purchase of alternative quantities of a good. If one accepts the arguments presented in this section, there are profound implications concerning the wisdom of relying on competitive markets in health system financing and medical care delivery. Some of these applications are provided in Section 3.3.

In the process, we will question six of the assumptions of the competitive economic model presented earlier:

Assumption 4. A person is the best judge of his or her own welfare.

Assumption 5. Consumers have sufficient information to make good choices.

Assumption 6. Consumers know, with certainty, the results of their consumption decisions.

Assumption 7. Individuals are rational.

Assumption 8. Individuals reveal their preferences through their actions.

Assumption 9. Social welfare is based solely on individual utilities, which in turn are based solely on the goods and services consumed.

3.2.1 Social Welfare and Consumer Choice: A Syllogism

As we saw in Section 2.1.4, it is typically argued that an economic system that allows for consumer choice will, subject to some caveats,[6] result in Pareto optimality. Then, if society can reach some agreement on its

---

5. Other economists have also employed Dr. Pangloss in their critiques of contemporary economics. See, for example, Culyer (1982).

6. The primary caveat is that externalities are unimportant. That is why economists often say that the presence of important yet uncorrected externalities results in "market failure."

social welfare function, redistribution can be implemented in ways that will maximize social welfare.

In this chapter, we will make the assumption that such a redistribution does occur. (Problems with this assumption were introduced in Section 2.2.2, which concerned positive externalities of consumption, and Chapter 5 will elaborate on those problems.) By doing so, we are implicitly assuming that reaching Pareto optimality will ultimately lead to the maximization of social welfare. This allows us to explicitly examine the assumptions under which allowing consumers to choose in the marketplace will be best for society as a whole.

With this assumption in hand, we can form the following syllogism: If

A. Social welfare is maximized when individual utilities are maximized,

and

B. Individual utilities are maximized when people are allowed to choose,

then:

C. Social welfare is maximized when people are allowed to choose.

This is obviously a strong conclusion because it implies that the type of consumer choice brought about by market competition will result, as Dr. Pangloss would say, in the best of all possible worlds. In the health field, the argument would provide strong ammunition for the superiority of competitive approaches. But if either proposition A or proposition B does not hold, then such a conclusion about the superiority of competition is not warranted. In the next section, we will attempt to cast serious doubt about the validity of both propositions A and B—first proposition B, and then A. Because proposition B encompasses five of the assumptions on which the advantages of competition are based, most of the emphasis will be on it.

3.2.2 Are Individual Utilities Maximized When People Are Allowed to Choose?

One of the basic tenets of market competition is that people are best off when they are allowed to make choices. If, instead, some entity such as government makes the choices for them, it is extremely unlikely that consumers will fare as well; each person is different, and it would seem to be impossible for an outsider to appreciate an individual's exact desires. True, sometimes people are poorly informed about a particular good or service and must rely on the advice of an *agent* such as a physician. But even then, they still choose whether to seek that advice, as well as the particular agent from whom the advice is sought.

In a world such as ours, where high-paid consultants abound and access to more information seems to be the key to success, it is noteworthy that economists often consider an individual consumer to be the world's greatest expert in one particular area. That area, of course, is what he or she wants. This viewpoint is nicely stated by economist Friedrich Hayek (1945), another of the founders of modern competitive theory:

> Today it is almost heresy to suggest that scientific knowledge is not the sum of all knowledge. But a little reflection will show that there is beyond question a body of very important but unorganized knowledge which cannot possibly be called scientific . . . : the knowledge of the particular circumstances of time and place. It is with respect to this that practically every individual has some advantage over all others in that he possesses unique information of which beneficial use might be made, but of which use can be made only if the decisions depending on it are left to him or are made with his active cooperation. . . . If we agree that the economic problem of society is mainly one of rapid adaptation to changes in the particular circumstances of time and place, it would seem to follow that the ultimate decisions must be left to the people who are familiar with these circumstances. (pp. 521–22, 534)

This is indeed a persuasive argument. Nevertheless, this section will attempt to demonstrate that, at least in the health area, allowing people to make their own choices does not necessarily make people best off.

The belief that consumers will find themselves in a best-off position when they have sovereignty over their market choices is based on several assumptions in the traditional competitive model:

- A person is the best judge of his or her own welfare (Assumption 4).
- People have the ability to make choices that are in their best interest:
  — Consumers have sufficient information to make good choices (Assumption 5).
  — Consumers know, with certainty, the results of their consumption decisions (Assumption 6).
  — Individuals are rational (Assumption 7).
- Individuals reveal their preferences through their actions (Assumption 8).

Is a Person the Best Judge of His or Her Own Welfare?

The first question that needs to be addressed when considering whether sovereignty is best for consumers is whether consumers are the foremost authority of what is in their best interest. As Hayek pointed out, in many instances they unquestionably are. Nevertheless, they may not be in all areas. If, in some instances, consumers are not the best judge of what is in their interest, then choices in such areas can perhaps be relegated to some other entity.

Of the several assumptions that we question in this chapter, this is perhaps the most difficult because of the seeming impossibility for empirical testing. There is, obviously, no direct source of information on what is best for a particular person. Consequently, there is no way of objectively testing who—the individual or some other entity—is the better agent for obtaining what is best for the person. We must therefore rely on indirect methods to further our inquiry.

To demonstrate that the individual is not necessarily the best judge, we will examine how society goes about making allocation decisions about particular goods and services. What we will try to show is that most societies set rules that are explicitly designed to thwart the sanctity of individual choice.

Below is a list of practices that a libertarian—that is, a person who believes in the sanctity of individual sovereignty—would likely believe should be left up to the individual rather than be proscribed by society:

- personal use of narcotic drugs;
- gambling;
- prostitution;
- riding a motorcycle without a helmet;
- selling one's own organs; and
- suicide.

This list was chosen specifically because these are all decisions that mainly affect the individual in question rather than others. Other illegal activities, such as requiring one's child to work rather than go to school, were left out because they have a direct negative effect on someone other than the decision maker. In the first three examples, there may be some indirect externalities—for example, drug use or gambling leading to more robberies, or prostitution leading to more sexually transmitted diseases. But these are indirect consequences, and regardless, the last three would result in harm almost entirely to the individual.[7]

Why would society act in a way to abridge individual choice when consumer theory indicates that people can and do make welfare maximizing choices themselves? Robert Frank (1985) suggests an interesting possibility: people are overly concerned with their status and will make the wrong economic, social, and/or moral decisions in order to enhance this status. One way that young people might do this is to try to "look cool," for instance, by smoking, using drugs, not wearing seat belts or helmets, or spending $200 on a pair of athletic shoes. Some of these practices are easy to outlaw, although rules against them cannot necessarily be

---

7. It is true that there is an indirect effect on others in that health costs might be higher, but this is not the primary reason why these activities are illegal.

enforced. But even the more vexing behaviors, such as excessive spending on status-building clothing, are not beyond society's grip. Many public schools are now adopting uniform requirements as a way of reducing the negative manifestations of status seeking.

Even adults might be lured by bad long-run choices. Frank suggests that this tends to manifest itself when adults make shortsighted decisions to obtain quick income in order to have money available to spend on consumables that ostensibly are status enhancing (e.g., fancy clothing or cars or new electronic equipment). It seems likely that people engaging in heavy gambling are doing it not in order to make money to save for their children's college education, but rather, to go on a spending spree. Similarly, one would imagine that an individual who sells one of his or her internal organs is doing so for reasons that, an objective observer would say, are not in that individual's best interest.

But trying to cut down on harmful status seeking does not seem to fully account for laws abridging personal choice. There is nothing status-raising about going to Mexico to purchase a supposed cure for cancer. Thus, another reason for paternalistic laws that limit individual choice is that some types of spending decisions are simply a waste of money: society is protecting people against their own foolishness.

A related reason for paternalism—one that is frequently cited in the health field—is that there are "experts" who know more than consumers, and can thus make better choices. In this regard, Tibor Scitovsky (1976) has written,

> The economist's traditional picture of the economy resembles nothing so much as a Chinese restaurant with its long menu. Customers choose from what is on the menu and are assumed always to have chosen what most pleases them. That assumption is unrealistic, not only of the economy, but of Chinese restaurants. Most of us are unfamiliar with nine-tenths of the entrees listed; we seem invariably to order either the wrong dishes or the same old ones. Only on occasions when an expert does the ordering do we realize how badly we do on our own and what good things we miss. (pp. 149–50)

It would seem clear, then, that society does not always judge people's decisions to be in their best interests. In making this judgment, society often acts to prevent people from engaging in some activity. The main pattern in this regard is that society often tells people what they cannot do; less often do we see situations in which people are told what they must do. This is certainly the case in health. People are told, for example, that they cannot purchase pharmaceutical drugs without a prescription. However, they are not told that they must take such drugs.

Do People Have the Ability to Make Choices That Are in Their Best Interest?

As noted above, for the answer to this question to be affirmative, three other questions must be answered in the affirmative: Do consumers have enough information to make good choices? Do consumers know the results of their consumption decisions? and Are individuals rational?

Do Consumers Have Enough Information To Make Good Choices?

Even if people know what they want and can pursue it in a rational manner, another impediment can stand in the way of people's best choices for themselves—that is, insufficient information about various alternatives.

Economic theory pins much responsibility on the role of good consumer information. Consumers, for example, need good information to make utility-maximizing product choices, firms need good information to choose a product niche and economically obtain the necessary inputs to maximize profits, and workers need good information to obtain a job that jointly satisfies the desire for professional satisfaction and good wages.

Indeed, in the health area, one frequently reads journal articles by economists calling for more information. To give one example, in discussing whether there is a welfare loss associated with excess amounts of health insurance—a topic considered in Section 3.3.1—Roger Feldman and Bryan Dowd (1993) state that, "if there is an inefficiently low level of information in medical care markets, the solution is to inform consumers, not to insure them fully" (p. 199).

The standard rallying cry to allow for more competition so long as there is better information is not viewed sympathetically by some noneconomist observers. Sociologist David Mechanic (1990) has stated,

> To many economists, purchasing health care is fundamentally no different than purchasing carrots or cameras, and many of the uncertainties or imperfections of medical care markets can be accounted for by "information costs," the residual category of economic analysis that seemingly explains away many of the core concerns of the other social sciences. (p. 93)

The question we need to consider, then, is whether people have enough information available to them to make the right choices. This obviously depends on the type of health service being considered, and unfortunately, very little research is available on the subject. Most work in this area has examined physicians.

An intriguing debate on how much information consumers need was carried out in a now almost legendary 1977 conference sponsored by the U.S. Federal Trade Commission.[8] Mark Pauly (1978) argued that we need to consider separately three kinds of services:

- those purchased relatively frequently by the typical household;
- those provided frequently by a physician, but used infrequently by a patient; and
- services that even a physician provides infrequently.

The first group would include pediatric care, dental care, prescription drugs, and the like. The second would include most surgical procedures, and the third, unusual and experimental procedures. Although Pauly thought that current information should be sufficient for consumers to make good choices in the first category of services, he estimated that three-fourths of expenditures would fall into the second and third categories.

In another conference paper, Frank Sloan and Roger Feldman (1978) argued that "standard [economic] theory does not require that *everyone* possess perfect information—only that there be a sufficient number of marginal consumers both able to assess output and willing to seek it out at its lowest price." They quote Pauly in this regard:

> I know even less about the works of a movie camera than I know about my own organs; yet I feel fairly confident in purchasing a camera for a given price as long as I know that there are at least a few experts in the market who are keeping sellers reasonably honest. (Feldman and Sloan 1978, 61)

Uwe Reinhardt (1978) criticized this viewpoint by presenting two sets of "rather bewildering" sets of specifications for stereo amplifiers. He then notes:

> Consider now a consumer without knowledge of electronics, with an only moderately sensitive ear. It can be wondered how our consumer would necessarily be driven to select the right model from these and other models *for his or her particular circumstances* simply because true experts in the market have established reasonable prices for these models, *given these experts' predilections and circumstances*. Chances are that our consumer would rely on expert advice in making the selection; chances are that the *vendor* would offer much advice freely; and chances are that the consumer will take home a model that may not be the most appropriate for his or her particular circumstances, especially if the vendor is overstocked on a particular model or

---

8. Ten years later, the Summer 1988 issue of the *Journal of Health Politics, Policy and Law* was devoted to a follow-up of these issues. The Fall 1989 issue of the journal included a critique of some aspects of this follow-up.

if profit margins differ among models. It could happen even to an economist! (Reinhardt 1978, 165)[9]

There has been some empirical research on how consumers go about trying to collect information on the alternatives they face in the health market. A number of fairly old studies have found relatively little evidence of "consumerism" in the health area, with one physician observer sardonically noting that consumers "devote more effort selecting their Halloween pumpkin than they do choosing their physician."[10] A more recent study, by Thomas Hoerger and Leslie Howard (1995), examined how pregnant women search for a prenatal care provider. The sample included women from Florida who gave birth in 1987. Women who believed that they had a choice of prenatal providers were asked, "Before you selected your actual prenatal care provider, did you seriously consider using another prenatal care provider?" If they answered that in the affirmative, they were further queried, "Did you actually speak with or have an appointment with another prenatal care provider?" Curiously, only 24 percent of the respondents seriously considered using another provider, and only 14 percent actually had contact with another provider. The authors conclude:

> This amount of search is surprisingly low, given the importance of childbirth, the ample opportunity for choice, and the relative surplus of information about prenatal care providers compared to providers of other physician services. Recall that we expected the choice of prenatal care providers to establish a benchmark or *upper bound* on the extent of search for other physician services. (Hoerger and Howard 1995, 341, italics added)

Interestingly, experience from previous births did not explain the results. For most women, the birth examined was the first child; and furthermore, women with previous births were more likely to search for a provider than those who were having their first child.

Thus, the little we know on the topic indicates that consumers often do not seek out information in order to choose a physician. But there is another, equally important question that needs to be addressed: Are consumers able to successfully use the information that *is* made available to them? Judith Hibbard and Edward Weeks (1989a,b) conducted studies of how information about physician fees affects consumers' knowledge levels and their use of services. Using data from random samples of state

---

9. This issue about what economists often call "asymmetric information" between the provider and patient will be taken up again in Chapter 4, where we consider supply-side issues in health economics.

10. This quotation, from Dr. Harvey Mandell, is from Hoerger and Howard (1995). The Hoerger and Howard article contains a good review of the literature on consumers' search for physicians.

government employees and Medicare beneficiaries in Oregon during the mid-1980s, the researchers divided sample members into experimental and control groups. The experimental group received a directory listing the fees for common procedures among area physicians, as well as a summary chart showing the ranges. Although receiving the directory resulted in increased knowledge levels among the government employees (but not the Medicare beneficiaries), the authors found that it did not result in changed behavior. The behaviors examined included asking about the costs of visits, procedures, tests, or medications; or changing physicians or insurance plans (Hibbard and Weeks 1989a). They also found that receipt of the information had no effect on costs per physician visit, the number of visits, or on annual health expenditures (Hibbard and Weeks 1989a). Although some of the sample had multiple insurance policies that would have covered the cost-sharing requirements associated with higher physician charges, the authors found that cost information had no effect even on those sample members who claimed costs to be a financial burden (Hibbard and Weeks 1989b).

The increased importance of managed care and capitation in the U.S. health system brings with it many challenges for consumers. To make the most appropriate choices about health plans, consumers need to understand such concepts as primary care gatekeeping, financial incentives to providers, and other plan characteristics that affect the type of care patients receive. Unfortunately, there is little evidence that consumers do understand these concepts.

When surveyed, most consumers do not understand the difference between fee-for-service medicine and managed care plans, even at a rudimentary level (Isaacs 1996). This finding is reinforced by a similar one—that most consumers believe that the health plan they choose is not an important determinant of the quality of care they will receive (Hibbard, Sofaer, and Jewett 1966; Jewett and Hibbard 1996). Such a belief indicates a lack of awareness of the many levers health plans have available to them to affect the types and quantity of services provided to plan members.

One important, relatively new area in which consumers will need to be skilled at using information is "report cards" on their health plans. People may obtain these report cards from their employer, and then are supposed to choose a health plan by weighing such factors as quality, convenience, flexibility, and costs.

At the time of writing, there is no one standard report card format. Passage of comprehensive health reform legislation in the United States during the early 1990s would have spurred the development of consistent information of this type. It is not clear, however, that the market will quickly come up with a standard report card. Consumers should easily understand some of the data items on early iterations of these report cards, such as satisfaction levels. But other elements will be more problematic. It is not clear, for example, that consumers will know how to make effective use of information on utilization rates for alternative services, or that they will understand the relative importance of survival rates from high-incidence versus low-incidence procedures.

Most of the current quality measures on report cards are based on the Health Plan Employer Data and Information Set (HEDIS), sponsored by the National Committee on Quality Assurance. HEDIS includes various measures of health plan performance in such areas as provision of preventive care to members and the appropriateness of care for particular problems, as well as patient satisfaction. When asked what they would expect to learn from different HEDIS measures, consumers typically ignore the data elements that they do not understand—which tend to be the "objective" measures of quality such as various utilization rates. Similarly, they overinterpret what can be learned from simple satisfaction data, the one element that they do tend to understand. Hibbard and Jewett (1997) report that,

> Interestingly, consumers perceive that patient ratings of overall quality give more information about the monitoring and follow-up of a condition than do the HEDIS indicators designed specifically for this purpose (such as rates of eye examinations among diabetic members, asthma hospitals, and low-birthweight infants). . . . These findings suggest that consumers are unsure of what many indicators are intended to tell them. (pp. 224–25)

They further note that,

> Great expectations are being placed on consumers. Without informed consumer choice, market reform is threatened, and consumers' interests are undermined. Yet little attention is given to help consumers understand the new environment, their role in it, or even how to interpret or use the new information sources. If informed consumer choice is to work, we must move beyond information dissemination to education about quality-of-care information, the new health environment, and the critical role for consumers in ensuring quality. (p. 227)

It is therefore not surprising that a study of managed care in 15 representative communities during 1995 concluded that, although there is much competition on the basis of price, "in general, there was almost no competition on the basis of measured and reported technical quality process or outcome measures" (Miller 1996, 116).

How, then, can consumers get the information that they need? In a study of this problem, Marc Rodwin (1996) concludes that this can come about only through a large-scale organized consumer movement:

Effective consumer protection requires organized consumer groups that are strong enough to make plans respond to their interests. . . . Consumers need organized groups to ensure the presence of and to monitor traditional government oversight; to help define policies and practices within managed care organizations; to monitor the performance of managed care organizations and private accrediting groups; to marshal political resources; and to form strategic alliances. (p. 112)

Currently, no such effort has been undertaken in the health area.[11]

Do Consumers Know the Results of Their Consumption Decisions?

Another concern about whether consumers can make appropriate choices involves a special characteristic in health known as the "counterfactual." Counterfactual questions are those that are hypothetical in a special way: they concern what would have happened if history had been different. To illustrate, some economists have tried to determine how quickly the western United States would have developed in the absence of railways (Fogel 1964; Fishlow 1965). Questions such as these can never be answered with certainty because there is no way to ascertain the future if the past activities are (artificially) altered.

The health area poses many counterfactual questions. Suppose a person seeks care from a primary care physician and tries to determine what he or she learned from the experience. It turns out to be very difficult for the person to determine whether he or she made the right decision in seeking care from that provider, because to do so would involve answering several counterfactual questions, such as:

- "Would the problem have gone away if I had left it untreated?"
- "What would have happened if I had sought the care of a specialist instead of a primary care physician?"
- "Would the result have been different if I had seen a different primary care physician than the one I sought?"

In this regard, Burton Weisbrod (1978) has written that,

For ordinary goods, the buyer has little difficulty in evaluating the counterfactual—that is, what the situation will be if the good is not obtained. Not so for the bulk of health care. . . . Because the human physiological system

---

11. Perhaps the closest activities currently available are state counseling programs, funded by the federal government, that provide counseling, seminars, and other information, largely to Medicare beneficiaries who need advice on the purchase of private insurance to supplement Medicare (including HMO coverage), Medicaid, or long-term care coverage, or assistance in handling claims forms. These programs, however, are quite small in scope, with an average expenditure of only 65 cents per Medicare beneficiary per year, and do not focus on the working-age population (McCormack et al. 1996).

is itself an adaptive system, it is likely to correct itself and deal effectively with an ailment, even without any medical care services. Thus, a consumer of such services who gets better after the purchase does not know whether the improvement was because of, or even in spite of, the "care" that was received. Or if no health care services are purchased and the individual's problem becomes worse, he is generally not in a strong position to determine whether the results would have been different, and better, if he had purchased certain health care. And the consumer, not being a medical expert, may learn little from experience or from friends' experience . . . because of the difficulty of determining whether the counterfactual to a particular type of health care today is the same as it was the previous time the consumer, or a friend, had "similar" symptoms. The noteworthy point is not simply that it is difficult for the consumer to judge quality before the purchase . . . but that it is difficult even after the purchase. (p. 52)

Weisbrod concludes that "when buyers have difficult quality-evaluation problems, the theorem of economics that more information . . . is always preferred to less need not hold" (p. 54).

Are Individuals Rational?

We must also consider whether consumers act rationally. This is really a very different question than whether people are the best judge of their own welfare. Even if people know what will make them best off, it does not necessarily mean that they will make choices that are consistent with this knowledge.

Before addressing this, we need to consider the meaning of "rational." Economists typically use a rather technical definition, whereby a person is rational if his or her other choices are consistent and transitive.[12] Consistency can be thought of as meaning that, if a person faces the exact same circumstances more than one time, the person will make the same choice. Transitive means that if a consumer prefers (and therefore chooses) good A over good B, and good B over good C, then he or she would also prefer (and choose) good A over C.

Although this definition will not be employed here, it is noteworthy that research on people's behavior has found numerous situations in which people do not act rationally in the economic sense. (See Thaler 1992, for a book full of such "anomolies.") Tversky and Kahneman (1981) provide a health example. In one experiment, they took two groups of people, asking the first,

Imagine that the U.S. is preparing for the outbreak of an unusual Asian disease, which is expected to kill 600 people. Two alternative programs to

---

12. See, for example, Mishan (1982).

combat the disease have been proposed. Assume that the exact scientific estimate of the consequences are as follows: If Program A is adopted, 200 people will be saved. If Program B is adopted, there is a 1/3 probability that 600 people will be saved, and 2/3 probability that no people will be saved. Which of the two programs would you favor? (Tversky and Kahneman 1981, p. 453)

Under this scenario, 72 percent chose Program A, indicating that they exhibit so-called risk-averse behavior.

The second group of people was asked the same question, but with two changes: "If Program C is adopted 400 people will die. If Program D is adopted there is a 1/3 probability that nobody will die, and 2/3 probability that 600 people will die" (Tversky and Kahneman 1981, p. 453). Under this scenario, 78 percent chose Program D. The authors conclude,

> The preferences . . . illustrate a common pattern: choices involving gains are often risk averse and choices involving losses are often risk taking. However, it is easy to see that the two problems are effectively identical. The only difference between them is that the outcomes are described in problem 1 by the number of lives saved and in problem 2 by the number of lives lost. The change is accompanied by a pronounced shift from risk aversion to risk taking. We have observed this reversal in several groups of respondents, including university faculty and physicians. (Tversky and Kahneman 1981, p. 453)

The economic definition is not terribly useful to us because the term "rationality" means much more than that. Here, we propose that rationality be thought of as indicating *reasonable* behavior.[13] An example will help illustrate what we mean by this term. If an adult in the United States smokes cigarettes, we do not necessarily regard this as irrational. This is because there are several potentially reasonable bases for some people to smoke. They may derive pleasure from smoking, they may feel that it enhances their image among a certain social group, or perhaps most importantly, they may be physically addicted. Thus, smoking can be a reasonable decision if the benefits outweigh the various costs. Now suppose that such a person also claims that smoking does nothing to

---

13. Not all economists would agree with this. In fact, some practitioners have tried to show that many seemingly self-destructive human behaviors, such as drug addiction and even suicide, are the result of utility-maximizing decisions! There is a body of literature—known as "rational addiction" theory—that purports to show drug and alcohol addiction to be consistent with rationality. Becker and Murphy (1988), for example, claim that "addictions, even strong ones, are usually rational in the sense of involving forward-looking maximization with *stable preferences*" (p. 675, emphasis added), and that even though unhappy people often become addicted, "they would be even more unhappy if they were prevented from consuming the addictive goods" (p. 691). Such a viewpoint flies in the face not only of common sense, but of the professional opinions of the vast majority of health professionals. Thus, this view of rationality is rejected here.

harm health, and cannot point to a heavy-smoking aunt who lived to age 93 and died peacefully in her sleep. If the person is even minimally educated, that sort of behavior should be viewed as irrational because it is not based on reason. To deny that cigarette smoking can harm one's health simply does not make sense.

Economists, in contrast to social scientists in other disciplines, sometimes suppose that consumers must be rational and must therefore act to maximize their utility. But that supposition would seem to be false. In this regard, Harvey Leibenstein (1976) has noted that "the idea of utility maximization must contain the possibility of choice under which utility is not maximized" (p. 8). Similarly, Lester Thurow (1983) writes,

> Revealed preferences . . . is just a fancy way of saying that individuals do whatever individuals do, and whatever they do, economists will call it "utility maximization." Whether individuals buy good A or good Y they are still rational individual utility maximizers. By definition, there is no such thing as an individual who does not maximize utility. But if a theory can never be wrong, it has no content. It is merely a tautology. (pp. 217–18)

This book is not the appropriate place for a thorough consideration of the validity of the rationality assumption. Indeed, much of the field of psychology, and some of the sociology literature, has been devoted to this issue. We will discuss only one such issue here because it has been well researched in the field of social psychology but only touched on by economists—cognitive dissonance.

The theory of cognitive dissonance concerns a central aspect of human behavior—self-justification or rationalization. As explained by Elliot Aronson (1972),

> Basically, cognitive dissonance is a state of tension that occurs when an individual simultaneously holds two cognitions (ideas, attitudes, beliefs, opinions) that are psychologically inconsistent. . . . Because [its] occurrence . . . is unpleasant, people are motivated to reduce it. . . . To hold two ideas that contradict each other is to flirt with absurdity, and—as Albert Camus, the existentialist philosopher, has observed—man is a creature who spends his entire life in an attempt to convince himself that his existence is not absurd. (pp. 92–93)

Whether people act in a way that we might define as rational or irrational depends on how difficult it is to change the behavior in question versus the cognition. Smoking offers one of the best examples. Suppose that a person smokes but knows that smoking is very dangerous to health. This causes cognitive dissonance; how can you continue to do something that is so self-destructive? If the person is not addicted or has a particularly strong will, he or she may quit. But an addict or a weaker person will typically find it easier to change the cognition rather than the behavior, either by attributing more pleasure to smoking than is truly obtained, or by denying that it is dangerous (Aronson 1972). Although this latter type of behavior has been repeatedly confirmed and is certainly understandable, it would seem to be a violation of the English language to deem it as "rational."

Economists George Akerlof and William Dickens (1992) have used cognitive dissonance to explain various economic behaviors. Examples include explaining the choice of risky jobs, technological development, advertising, social insurance, and crime. Regarding social insurance, they write:

> If there are some persons who would simply prefer not to contemplate a time when their earning power is diminished, and if the very fact of saving for old age forces persons into such contemplations, there is an argument for compulsory old age insurance. . . . [They] may find it uncomfortable to contemplate their old age. For that reason they may make the wrong tradeoff, *given their own preferences*, between current consumption and savings for retirement. (p. 317, italics added)

Note that saving is what would make people best off in their own eyes, but they fail to do it anyway. Hence, society makes the decision to override individual choice by establishing social insurance programs—like Social Security and Medicare.

In summary, when cognitive dissonance is important, there is little reason to suppose that people will act in a rational manner—that is, make decisions that truly maximize their utility.

Do Individuals Reveal Their Preferences Through Their Actions?

Amartya Sen (1982, 1987, 1992) has written a number of persuasive essays and books on this issue. The basic problem concerns an issue addressed earlier, in Section 2.2—interdependencies in people's utility functions. If people make their choices based not only on their own preferences but on the preferences of others as well, then these choices will not necessarily reflect their personal preferences. This becomes extremely important because it casts doubt on the conventional meaning of demand curves, which purport to show the marginal utility that people obtain from additional units of consumption.

This viewpoint is supported by Frank (1985), who writes,

> The economist's most favored methods for measuring benefits are all based on the theory of revealed preference. This theory says that when a person buys one combination of goods when he could have bought another, he reveals by

his action that he prefers the first combination to the second. This is a truism where individually defined preferences are concerned. But it is false when there are important interdependencies between people. (pp. 205–6)

Sen and Frank both illustrate this point by bringing up the well-known "Prisoners' Dilemma." In this example, two prisoners are each faced with the decision either to confess or not to confess to a crime for which they are jointly guilty. If one confesses and the other does not, the former goes free and the latter receives a long prison term (say, 30 years). If both confess, they receive a much shorter term (5 years). If neither confesses, they can be prosecuted only for a lesser crime and would receive only 1 year in prison.

It would seem to be rational for each prisoner to confess. Imagine that you and I are the prisoners, and suppose first that you confess. If I confess, I go to prison for 5 years, versus 30 years if I do not confess. Now suppose that you do not confess. If I confess, I get no prison time, versus 1 year if I do not. Thus, it would seem to be in my interest (and therefore yours since you face the same schedule of penalties as I) to confess. But this, of course, is not the case. If we both confess, we get 5 years of prison; but if neither of us confesses, we serve only a year.

Sen points out that this outcome can be arrived at if each prisoner tries to mimic the preferences of the *other* prisoner, rather than himself. Suppose I want to minimize your prison term. Knowing that you are rational and would confess, I would not confess, and in that way you would get no prison (and I would get 30 years). And if you act the same way—in my interests rather than in your own—we will jointly reach the optimal strategy. Neither of us will confess, and we will each get only 1 year in prison.

In this regard, Sen (1982) writes:

Each [prisoner] is assumed to be self-centered and interested basically only in his own prison term, and the choice of non-confession follows *not* from calculations based on this welfare function, but from following a moral code of behaviour suspending the rational calculus. . . . And it is this difference that is inimical to the revealed preference approach to the study of human behaviour. . . . The interest in the prisoners' dilemma lies not in the fiction which gives the problem its colour, but in the existence of a strictly dominant strategy for each person which together produce a strictly inferior outcome for all. . . . The essence of the problem is that if both prisoners behave *as if* they are maximizing a different welfare function from the one that they actually have, they will both end up being better off even in terms of their *actual* welfare function. . . . This is where the revealed preference approach goes off the rails altogether. The behavior pattern that will make each better off in terms of their real preferences is not at all the behaviour pattern that will *reveal* those real preferences. Choices that reveal individual preferences may be quite inefficient for achieving welfare of the group. . . . I would argue that the philosophy of the revealed preference approach essentially underestimates the fact that man is a social animal and his choices are not rigidly bound to his own preferences only. I do not find it difficult to believe that birds and bees and dogs and cats do reveal their preferences by their choice; it is with human beings that the proposition is not particularly persuasive. An act of choice for this social animal is, in a fundamental sense, always a social act. (pp. 65–66)

On perhaps a less abstract level, Sen argues that much human behavior that we witness flies in the face of the notion that your actions indicate your personal preferences. He does this by distinguishing two concepts, sympathy and commitment. A person who acts on feelings of sympathy is indeed showing his personal preferences through his actions; you feel better if you help. Commitment, however, is different; you would rather do something else but you do not because you are committed to a particular cause. Sen uses recycling as an example. He argues that people recycle not because they enjoy it or because they believe that their own recycling behavior will make a marked difference in the cleanliness of the environment, nor do they think that their own actions will convince anyone else to do it, but they do it anyway because of their commitment to a cleaner environment. He summarizes this point, noting that "one way of defining commitment is in terms of a person choosing an act that he believes will yield a lower level of personal welfare to him than an alternative that is also available to him" (Sen 1982, 92). Sen notes further that this concept "drives a wedge between personal choice and personal welfare, [but] much of traditional economic theory relies on the identity of the two" (p. 94).

People's actions, at times, therefore seem to be motivated by things other than selfishness, and thus, the choices one observes do not necessarily indicate the level of welfare derived by the individual or by society. (In this regard, Sen [1982] writes, "The *purely* economic man is indeed close to being a social moron" [p. 99].) But the results of this behavior can go in either direction: either choosing something that enhances social but not personal welfare (e.g., commitment); or choosing not to help others when it would be personally beneficial to do so. S. K. Nath (1969) provides a useful example of the latter behavior.

Suppose we observe a person *not* giving to a charity aimed at improving the health of the poor. Using revealed preference, one would conclude that the person would rather have something else—the good or service purchased with the money that could have been spent on the charity. This might not be the case, however. It may be that the person would benefit from providing such a donation because his utility function contains an element encompassing the health of the poor. But he may believe that his contribution will not be of much help because others are not compelled to follow suit.[14] Thus, the person would like the poor to have better access to health services, but this is not evidenced by his or her market behavior. Nath states that there is a "fallacy in the assumption than an individual's welfare function coincides with his utility function as revealed by his market choices. This is a very common fallacy in economic writings" (p. 141).

What we have tried to show in Section 3.2.2 is that proposition B in the syllogism presented above—that individual utilities are maximized when people are allowed to choose—often may not be met in the health area. The next section examines the validity of the other proposition that must be met in order for consumer choice to result, of necessity, in what is best for society.

3.2.3 Is Social Welfare Maximized When Individual Utilities Are Maximized?

This section examines proposition A of the syllogism presented earlier, that social welfare is maximized when individuals maximize their own utility. This is essentially the same thing as Assumption 9 from Table 1.1:

Assumption 9. Social welfare is based solely on individual utilities, which in turn are based solely on the goods and services consumed.

Recall that in this chapter, we are making the assumption that society can and does redistribute income. (Problems with this assumption can be found earlier in Section 2.2.2, which concerned externalities of consumption, and in Chapter 5.) This allows us to examine explicitly the advantages of allowing for consumer choice in the health market without worrying about issues of equity.

Although the proposition that social welfare is based solely on individuals' welfare is a philosophical issue and cannot be proved true or false, there are two reasons to question its validity. The first of these arguments is also from Sen (1982, 1987, 1992), who disputes this notion that individual welfare is the only legitimate component of social welfare.

---

14. This is called the "free-rider effect." In this case, I would like to give to charity if it makes a difference to the poor, but my contribution, by itself, will make almost no difference. If everyone contributes, it will make a difference, of course. I may realize that the poor would be just about as well off if I were a free rider, that is, if I did not contribute but everyone else did. The problem is that, if everyone acts this way, little will be contributed to the poor.

He calls such a philosophy "welfarism," which "is the view that the only things of intrinsic value for ethical calculation and evaluation of states of affairs are individual utilities" (Sen 1987, p. 40). Sen's arguments, which span several books, are too lengthy to be properly summarized here. One of the reasons that Sen rejects the welfarist approach is that it does not allow us to distinguish between different *qualities* of utility. An example he gives is that, if you get pleasure from my unhappiness, that counts as much under the welfarist approach as anything else. In contrast, one might believe that a society should devote its resources to meeting somewhat more lofty desires. Another reason is that the concept of individual welfare does not seem to be well captured simply by the goods you have; other aspects of life, such as freedom, would also seem to be important. In this regard, Robin Hahnel and Michael Albert (1990) point out that conventional theory would make you equally well off if you are *assigned* a bundle of goods, versus a situation in which you *choose* the bundle. It does not take much introspection to realize that the latter may indeed result in higher utility.

A second reason to doubt that social welfare is not the sum of individual welfare is brought up by Frank (1985), who notes that much of what individuals seek out is status or rank. But these are relative things; if my status goes up, yours goes down by definition. This leads to a situation where people engage in consumption that does not add to the social welfare. For example, if I buy a fancy car, I get utility both from the various characteristics of the car, and from the fact that I have distinguished myself from you. Once you (and others like us) buy the car, the latter part of my utility is canceled out. Total utility (or social welfare) is thus lower than the sum of our individual utilities.

3.3 Implications for Health Policy

This chapter has attempted to show that there are various problems with inferring that the goods and services people demand in a competitive marketplace will necessarily make them best off. We have attempted to show that such a supposition is based on several assumptions whose fulfillment in the health area is open to serious question. This section provides a number of implications concerning the tools health economists use, and the issues they study.

3.3.1 Is Comprehensive National Health Insurance Necessarily Inefficient?

Some health economists have long contended that people in the United States and other developed countries are "overinsured," which results in a societal "welfare loss." That is, people have more insurance than is optimal for them or for society at large. To the noneconomist, this might seem like an odd belief, given the great concern about the number of uninsured people in the United States. In fact, nearly all economists would agree that a risk-averse[15] person would do better by purchasing fairly priced health insurance. Nevertheless, many economists contend that people with health insurance have too much coverage—that is, they do not have to pay enough of the costs of care out-of-pocket.

The Welfare Loss Argument

To better understand this argument, it is necessary to review a concept in insurance called *moral hazard*. Moral hazard exists when the possession of an insurance policy increases the likelihood of incurring a covered loss, and/or the size of a covered loss. The term dates back to the purchase of fire insurance in the nineteenth century. It was recognized that a business or person that had fire insurance on a property might be more likely to incur a loss—either by deliberately setting a fire (hence, "moral" hazard) or by being less diligent in ensuring that a fire would not start in the first place. A quotation from a textbook on fire insurance dating back to 1877 will give some flavor to the term:

> We cannot too earnestly impress upon [insurance] agents, everywhere, the necessity of care. The agent who contributes, by over-insurance or in any way, to an incendiary fire, *endangers the common safety and commits a crime against society.** Constant supervision and watchfulness, with a keen judgment of men and values, are necessary. . . . It must be borne in mind that companies sometimes lose as much in consequence of *the indifference of honest men . . . as by the designing villainy of those who do not scruple to apply the match.*
>
> *While overinsurance causes fires, a proper amount of insurance may prevent them by teaching a malicious vagabond that he cannot harm his enemy by burning his property, as the insurance company's interposition restores the loss. (Moore 1877, 18)

In the health area, the existence of moral hazard implies that people use more services when they are insured, or more fully insured. But as Mark Pauly (1968) pointed out in his famous essay on moral hazard, "the response of seeking more medical care with insurance than in its absence

---

15. A risk-averse person can be thought of as someone who prefers "a bird in the hand to two in the bush." The specific definition is that a person is risk averse if the marginal utility of additional income declines. In order words, if you make $30,000 a year, the last $1,000 you make brings about more utility than an additional $1,000 (that would make your income $31,000). It can be shown that such a person would generally want to buy insurance if the administrative or "loading" charges are small. For derivations of this, see Feldstein (1988) or Phelps (1992).

is a result not of moral perfidy, but of rational economic behavior" (p. 535). For a fully insured person, the cost of using an additional service will be shared by everyone who pays premiums. Thus, the person is likely to use more services than if he or she paid the full cost of the additional service.

In fact, the existence of moral hazard simply means that the demand curve for medical care slopes downward and to the right: People seek more services when their out-of-pocket payments are lower.

Despite the fact that moral hazard in medical care is an example of rational economic behavior, many economists are nevertheless troubled by its existence. This is because, when people are fully insured, they may demand services that only provide a small amount of benefit. But these services are likely to cost just as much as any other services. Thus, the benefits people derive from the purchase of these "marginal" services might be swamped by their cost.

In his article, Pauly tried to show that a country might be better off without compulsory, governmentally sponsored health insurance. This was in response to an article by Kenneth Arrow (1963b), who contended that government might be justified in providing such insurance out of tax dollars if a private market did not exist. It is instructive to examine Pauly's argument, as it will provide some useful guidance to the discussion that follows.

Suppose first that a person is uninsured, and has a 50 percent chance of staying well during a year, a 25 percent chance of being mildly sick, and a 25 percent chance of being very sick. Further suppose that his medical expenditures will be zero if he is well, $50 if he is mildly sick, and $200 if he is very sick. These expenditure levels are indicated by the vertical axis and vertical demand curves D_2' and D_3' in Figure 3.4, which are taken from Pauly's article. Consequently, the expected value of his annual medical costs will be $62.50 (.5 × $0 + .25 × $50 + .25 × $200). Now suppose that the person has health insurance that pays 100 percent of costs. Assume that he continues to use no services if he is not sick, but spends $150 (instead of $50) if he is mildly sick and $300 (instead of $200) if he is very sick. These expenditure levels are shown by the vertical axis and diagonal demand curves D_2 and D_3 in Figure 3.4. In this instance, the expected value of his annual costs will be $112.50 (.5 × $0 + .25 × $150 + .25 × 300).

Pauly's point is that the person might be better off with no insurance, and paying $62.50 a year out-of-pocket, than having government-sponsored insurance, and paying $112.50 in taxes. It is true that the person may have used more services with the insurance, but the services used

Figure 3.4 Pauly's Analysis of Welfare Loss

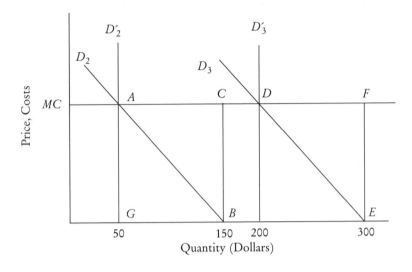

Source: Pauly, M. V. 1968. "The Economics of Moral Hazard: Comment." *American Economic Review* 58 (4): 531–37.

might not be of sufficient value to him to justify the additional $50 in expenditures.

Figure 3.4 can also be used to calculate the welfare loss of health insurance for this particular person. Recall that in conventional theory, a demand curve shows the marginal utility associated with alternative quantities purchased. A mildly sick person who is provided insurance coverage, and whose expenditures rise from $50 to $150, accrues benefits equal to the lower triangle *AGB*. However, the cost to society of producing these extra services is indicated by the square, *AGBC* (a constant marginal cost of producing services, *MC*, is assumed for convenience). Consequently, the upper triangle *ABC* provides an estimate of the welfare loss associated with health insurance. Adding this to the triangle *DEF*, which shows the welfare loss for very sick people, gives the total welfare loss. Pauly (1968) summarizes,

> [T]he inefficiency loss due to behavior under insurance, if that insurance were compulsory, would then be roughly measured by triangles ABC and DEF. These areas represent the excess that individuals do pay over what they would be willing to pay for the quantity of medical care demanded under insurance. Against this loss must be offset the utility gain from having these uncertain expenses insured, but the net change in utility from a compulsory purchase of this "insurance" could well be negative. (p. 534)

The existence of moral hazard that results from the possession of health insurance has made many economists conclude that there is a societal "welfare loss" associated with the ownership of too much health insurance. This is a very important conclusion; it implies that a society is not best off if its members have more health insurance than is deemed to be optimal. In a survey of U.S. and Canadian health economists conducted in 1989, 63 percent strongly or mildly agreed with the statement that health insurance causes societal welfare loss (Feldman and Morrisey 1990).

A number of researchers have computed the magnitude of this welfare loss for the United States as a whole.[16] One well-known set of estimates were calculated based on results of the RAND Health Insurance Experiment, which was conducted from 1974 through 1982. (This experiment is discussed in greater detail in Chapter 4.) In this study,[17] which constituted perhaps the most ambitious undertaking thus far in the field of health services research, individuals in six sites across the United States were randomly assigned to insurance plans that differed on the basis of patient coinsurance rates and some other factors. The effect of different coinsurance rates on annual expenditures is shown in the last column of Table 3.1. It was found that people who have to pay 95 percent of charges had annual expenditures that were 28 percent less than those who paid nothing. From a policy standpoint, perhaps more relevant is the finding that those facing a 25 percent coinsurance rate had expenditures that were 18 percent less than those with free care. Willard Manning et al. (1987) used these results to estimate a total welfare loss of $37 billion to $60 billion, which represented between 19 percent and 30 percent of total national health expenditures.

A more recent set of welfare loss estimates—also based on the RAND Health Insurance Experiment findings—come from a study by Feldman and Dowd (1991). This study provides a number of refinements over the previous one; in particular, it takes into account the fact that risk-averse individuals derive utility from being insured. It nevertheless concludes that the welfare loss associated with excess health insurance far outweighs the utility conveyed through owning insurance. Taking into account these conflicting components, the net welfare loss varied from $33 billion to $109 billion in 1984 dollars, depending on the assumptions employed,

---

16. The first such estimates were developed by Martin Feldstein, and published in Feldstein (1973).

17. See Phelps (1992) for a summary of this experiment and its findings. The most detailed description and summary of the study is contained in Newhouse et al. (1993).

Table 3.1 Findings from the RAND Health Insurance Experiment

Amount of Patient Coinsurance	Face-to-Face Visits	Outpatient Expenses (1984 $)	Admissions per 1,000 Population	Inpatient Dollars (1984 $)	Probability of Any Medical Care (%)	Probability of Any Inpatient Care (%)	Total Expenses (1984 $)	Adjusted Total Expenses (1984 $)
Free	4.55	340	128	409	86.8	10.3	749	750
25%	3.33	260	105	373	78.8	8.4	634	617
50%	3.03	224	92	450	77.2	7.2	674	573
95%	2.73	203	99	315	67.7	7.9	518	540

Source: Manning, W. G., et al. 1987. "Health Insurance and the Demand for Medical Care: Evidence from a Randomized Experiment." *American Economic Review* 77 (3): 259.

representing between 9 percent and 28 percent of health spending in the United States during that year.[18]

Critique of the Welfare Loss Argument

The argument supporting welfare loss from excess health insurance, and estimates of the magnitude of that loss, are based on the assumption that the demand curve shows the marginal utility that a person derives from an additional service. In Section 3.2, however, we questioned that interpretation. For a demand curve to represent the marginal utility of purchases, several assumptions have to be met: consumers must act rationally (Assumption 7), they must have sufficient information to make good choices (Assumption 5), and they must know what the results of their consumption decisions will be (Assumption 6).

In essence, what the welfare loss argument says is that consumers must be able to determine exactly how much an additional service is worth to them. Then, they compare this to its price to determine if it is worth their while to purchase the service. If people have insurance, the price they have to pay will be less; consequently, they will be more receptive to purchasing a service that conveys little utility. The difference between the cost of the service, and the utility received, equals the welfare loss from the purchase of that service.

The question we need to consider, then, is whether information is available that allows us to determine whether consumers can accurately estimate the marginal utility they receive from additional services. Fortunately, there is a method of testing this, although, as noted later, there are some problems with this method.

---

18. This calculation is based on figures provided in Levit et al. (1985).

It will be recalled that welfare loss occurs because consumers with health insurance have an incentive to purchase additional services (compared to what they would be purchasing without insurance) that provide little benefit to them. We can therefore examine whether this occurs by observing the kinds of services that consumers forgo when they are provided with less comprehensive insurance coverage. The results from the RAND Health Insurance study show that utilization will go down in the presence of coinsurance. And welfare loss theory tells us the types of services that ought to be forgone: those that provide relatively little utility.

The nature of this test is clarified in Figure 3.5, which is taken from an earlier work of the author (Rice 1992a). The horizontal line indicates the marginal cost of producing a service, which can be viewed as the cost to society—that is, the resources that have to be expended in providing a service. In a competitive market, that will also equal its price. The curved line, which is a demand curve, shows the marginal utility of each additional service. At a zero price—that is, with comprehensive insurance—the consumer will demand Q_0 services; the last such service provides very little utility.

Now suppose that there are two types of services—those that are highly effective (*HE*) and those that have low effectiveness (*LE*). Further suppose that the person no longer has health insurance, and his demand for care has declined from Q_0 to Q_1. It is clear from Figure 3.5 that the person would be expected to forgo the low-effectiveness service, *LE*, because its benefits are now outweighed by its costs. But service *HE* would still be purchased because its benefits exceed costs, even in the absence of insurance coverage. If people actually behaved as predicted, then we would have some confidence that the demand curve for medical care really shows the marginal utility consumers obtain from additional services. This, in turn, would provide support for the welfare loss estimates discussed above.

The problem with operationalizing this test, of course, is coming up with a way of determining the marginal utility consumers receive from a service. The proxy used here is a measure of the medical effectiveness of a service—as judged by medical experts. Although consumers and experts may differ in what they think is important, common sense tells us that consumers would prefer those services that are thought to be the most effective.

As part of the RAND study, Lohr et al. (1986) grouped services into categories based on their expected medical effectiveness:

Figure 3.5 Change in Demand for Services of Differing Effectiveness

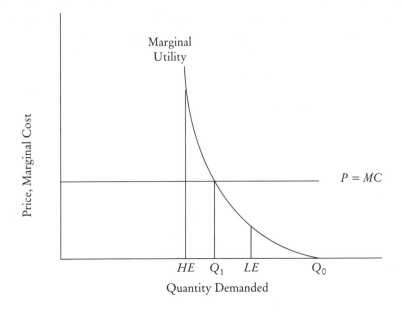

Source: Rice, T. 1992a. "An Alternative Framework for Evaluating Welfare Losses in the Health Care Market." *Journal of Health Economics* 11 (1): 88.

Group 1. Highly effective treatment by medical care system;
Group 2. quite effective treatment by medical care system;
Group 3. less effective treatment by medical care system; and
Group 4. medical care rarely effective or self-care effective.

The category into which a particular service falls is shown in Table 3.2, which is taken from the study.

The authors found that

> [C]ost-sharing was generally just as likely to lower use when care is thought to be highly effective as when it is thought to be only rarely effective, [nor] was there any obvious trend suggesting that cost-sharing would deter care seeking more as one moved "down" the effectiveness ranking. (p. S32)

They concluded that,

> [C]ost-sharing did not lead to rates of care seeking that were more "appropriate" from a clinical perspective. That is, cost-sharing did not seem to have a selective effect in prompting people to forgo care only or mainly in circumstances when such care probably would be of relatively little value. (p. S36)

Table 3.2 Medical Effectiveness Groupings in the Lohr et al. Study

Group 1: Highly Effective Treatment by Medical Care System
Medical care highly effective: acute conditions
Eyes—conjunctivitis
Otitis media, acute
Acute sinusitis
Strep throat
Acute lower respiratory infections (acute bronchitis)
Pneumonia
Vaginitis and cervicitis
Nonfungal skin infections
Trauma—fractures
Trauma—lacerations, contusions, abrasions
Medical care highly effective: acute or chronic conditions
Sexually transmitted disease or pelvic inflammatory disease
Malignant neoplasm, including skin
Gout
Anemias
Enuresis
Seizure disorders
Eyes—strabismus, glaucoma, cataracts
Otitis media, not otherwise specified
Chronic sinusitis
Peptic and nonpeptic ulcer disease
Hernia
Urinary tract infection
Skin—dermatophytoses
Medical care highly effective: chronic conditions
Thyroid disease
Diabetes
Otitis media, chronic
Hypertension and abnormal blood pressure
Cardiac arrythmias
Congestive heart failure
Chronic bronchitis, chronic obstructive pulmonary disease
Rheumatic disease (rheumatoid arthritis)
Group 2: Quite Effective Treatment by Medical Care System
Diarrhea and gastroenteritis (infectious)
Benign and unspecified neoplasm
Thrombophlebitis
Hemorrhoids
Hay fever (chronic rhinitis)
Acute middle respiratory infections (tracheitis, laryngitis)

Asthma
Chronic enteritis, colitis
Perirectal conditions
Menstrual and menopausal disorders
Acne
Adverse effects of medicinal agents
Other abnormal findings
Group 3: Less Effective Treatment by Medical Care System
Hypercholesterolemia, hyperlipidemia
Mental retardation
Peripheral neuropathy, neuritis, and sciatica
Ears—deafness
Vertiginous syndromes
Other heart disease
Edema
Cerebrovascular disease
Varicose veins of lower extremities
Prostatic hypertrophy, prostatitis
Other cervical disease
Lymphadenopathy
Vehicular accidents
Other injuries and adverse effects
Group 4: Medical Care Rarely Effective or Self-care Effective
Medical care rarely effective
Viral exanthems
Hypoglycemia
Obesity
Chest pain
Shortness of breath
Hypertrophy of tonsils or adenoids
Chronic cystic breast disease (nonmalignant)
Debility and fatigue (malaise)
Over-the-counter or self-care effective
Influenza (viral)
Fever
Headaches
Cough
Acute URI
Throat pain
Irritable colon
Abdominal pain
Nausea or vomiting
Constipation
Other rashes and skin conditions
Degenerative joint disease
Low back pain diseases and syndromes
Bursitis or synovitis and fibrositis or myalgia
Acute sprains and strains
Muscle problems

Source: Lohr, K. N., et al. 1986. "Effect of Cost Sharing on Use of Medically Effective and Less Effective Care." *Medical Care* 24: 9 (Supplement): Table 5.1, S33.

It is noteworthy that another component of the RAND study reached a similar conclusion regarding the effect of coinsurance on appropriate versus inappropriate hospitalization (Siu et al. 1986).

What does all this mean for the theory of welfare loss from excess health insurance?

> The Lohr et al. study shows that consumers who face cost-sharing reduce demand across-the-board, both for care that is highly effective and less effective. But the welfare loss argument rests on the supposition that the services forgone as a result of cost-sharing will be composed *entirely* of those that provide less utility; the Health Insurance Study clearly shows this is not the case. At the very least, only services providing the lower level of benefits (such as service [*LE*] in Fig. [3.5]) should be included in the welfare loss calculation. More generally, welfare loss calculations are hard to defend when it seems apparent that consumers cannot accurately value the benefits and costs of the medical services they consume. (Rice 1992a, 89)

This view—that patient demand curves show how much consumers buy at different prices, but not necessarily the utility they derive from such services—runs very much against the grain of conventional economic theory. It is not, however, unique among economists. One noteworthy example is from an article by Randall Ellis and Thomas McGuire (1993), who write,

> [W]e are skeptical that the observed demand can be interpreted as reflecting "socially efficient" consumption, [so] we interpret the demand curve in a more limited way, as an empirical relationship between the degree of cost sharing and quantity of use demanded by the patient. (p. 142)

As noted earlier, the argument against the welfare loss calculations depends in part on the existence of a close correspondence between consumer preferences and experts' opinion of the medical effectiveness of alternative services. Intuitively, one would imagine that there would be, since consumers would seem unlikely to want to use services that experts find to be of little value. A related issue needs to be raised, however: the validity of the Lohr et al. categories shown in Table 3.2. Feldman and Dowd (1993) note one example of a potential problem: medical care is considered to be highly effective for the treatment of strep throat, but rarely effective for throat pain (although self-care is effective). Others have noted that it seems odd to include chest pain in the category where medical care is rarely effective. These concerns are indeed important ones, but there is no other study on which we can rely to inform us about the issue at hand. Until there is, the Lohr et al. findings from the RAND study, in conjunction with the theory developed in Figure 3.5, must at the very minimum give us pause before accepting the conventional welfare loss methodology and estimates.

Where is the Waste in Medical Care?

In 1995, the United States almost topped the $1 trillion figure in health spending (the exact figure was $988.5 billion), with per capita expenditures exceeding $3,600 (Burner and Waldo 1995). This constituted 13.6 percent of national income, a figure about 30 percent higher than in any other country in the world (Schieber, Poullier, and Greenwald 1994).

Economists are often quick to point out that the $1 trillion and 14 percent figures do not provide any direct evidence that we are spending too much for medical care in the United States. Maybe, they contend, people really get more out of this high level of medical care spending that they would from spending it in alternative ways.[19] Although it is very difficult to disprove this contention, there is some circumstantial evidence to indicate that the United States is not getting as much out of this extra spending as it might expect.

Researchers have not been able to demonstrate that the high spending in the United States relative to other countries can be justified through evidence of better outcomes or higher quality. Although it is difficult to conduct valid cross-national studies of medical outcomes, what little evidence there is does not support the view that the United States is getting better outcomes for its money. Perhaps the most notable studies to date have been conducted by Roos et al. (1990), who have examined postsurgical mortality in the New England states versus Manitoba. The researchers divided procedures according to low, moderate, and high mortality, and looked at mortality rates 30 days, one year, and three years after surgery. After adjusting the best they could for case-mix differences, they found mortality rates to be lower in Manitoba for both low- and moderate-risk procedures, over all three time intervals. Thirty-day mortality rates were lower in New England for high-mortality procedures, but these differences subsided over time (Roos et al. 1992). The authors concluded that higher U.S. spending did not appear to manifest itself in better outcomes.

In addition, since the early work of John Wennberg and colleagues,[20] there has appeared to be much agreement among experts that many of the services provided are not medically necessary. Although little agreement has been reached on the magnitude of unnecessary services

---

19. As noted in Chapter 2, survey data show that about half of all Americans believe that the country spends too little on health (Blendon et al. 1995b).

20. Perhaps the best-known article is Wennberg and Gittlesohn (1982). For a thorough review of the literature through the mid-1980s, see Paul-Shaheen, Clark, and Williams (1987).

utilized, for some procedures it has been estimated to be as high as 30 percent (Leape 1989). As a result, probably the major research effort now being conducted by the health services research community at large is determining what services are and what services are not medically effective. This research is manifesting itself in two major ways: through the dissemination and use of practice guidelines for various medical conditions, and by "profiling" individual physicians' service provision rates. Managed care plans can then use the profiles in an attempt to assess physicians' medical decision making.

Where, then, is the waste in medical care? Under the traditional theory, the source of the waste is clear: patients demand too many services when they have complete or nearly complete insurance coverage. The alternative being presented here is that most of the waste is in the provision of services that do little or no good in improving the patients' health.[21] These alternative theories are not totally contradictory—some services could be deemed wasteful under both approaches (e.g., a person with complete insurance demands a service that brings him little utility, and that experts believe will have little or no effect on his or her health).

Nevertheless, the policy implications of the two approaches are *very* different. If one believes the conventional theory, policies should be enacted that make the user of services more sensitive to price. In contrast, if the problem is more in the area of the provision of services that are not useful, policies should target the provider of services.

The idea of pursuing supply-side rather than demand-side policies will be explored in greater detail in Chapter 4. The key point here is that most policies aimed at controlling costs in the United States—and practically all such policies in the rest of the world—are aimed at the supply side rather than the demand side. It is important to recognize that this contradicts conventional economic theory, in which consumers are the ones who should be in charge of deciding what services they should or should not receive because only they can measure the utility that such services will bring.

The supply-side policies that are now most common—putting physicians at risk through capitation or other forms of incentive reimbursement, utilization review, and technology controls and global budgets in many countries—are designed to influence the types of services provided, without consulting the patient. Thus, the policies are based, in part, on

---

21. Other writers have also advocated calculating welfare losses based on the provision of unnecessary services. See Phelps and Parente (1990), Phelps and Mooney (1992), Dranove (1995), and Phelps (1995b).

the belief that someone other than the consumer is the best judge of what medical services should be delivered.[22]

It is noteworthy that many analysts—economists as well as practitioners of other disciplines—believe that managed care strategies that are based on capitating health plans offer the best hope for controlling U.S. health costs. These strategies are aimed almost entirely at changing what services are provided by providers, rather than changing the demand by consumers. In fact, what is perhaps most noteworthy about the HMO approach to cost containment is that copayments are *lower* than the payments in fee-for-service medicine. If these strategies are designed to reduce waste, it would seem clear that the waste is thought to be generated through the provision of unnecessary services far more so than through excess demand by patients. And if this is true in the United States, it must be even more true in other developed countries, where, with very few exceptions, there are very few patient copayments, with almost all cost-control activities being focused on the providers of care.[23]

3.3.2 Should Patient Cost-Sharing Be Encouraged, or Should We Use Other Policies?

As indicated in Section 3.3.1, the thrust of the "welfare loss" literature is that more patient cost-sharing will be beneficial to society. This argument can be demonstrated by modifying Figure 3.4, to show how institution of a patient coinsurance rate would reduce the welfare loss of complete health insurance coverage. In Figure 3.4, the triangles ABC and DEF showed the original welfare loss from full insurance. With the institution of coinsurance, C, it would be cut to the sum of triangles AHI and DJK in Figure 3.6.

There is a danger in this sort of analysis, which has been noted by Robert Evans (1984): "The welfare burden is minimized when there is no insurance at all" (p. 49). If one takes this reasoning very far, it becomes apparent that the conventional analysis will always find that the country with higher patient cost-sharing requirements will have the more efficient health system (Reinhardt 1992). Thus, the U.S. system would be deemed more efficient than the Canadian system or any of a number of European systems, not because of a comparison of outcomes to costs, but rather simply from the fact that the U.S. imposes patient

---

22. This is not the only reason for such policies. Another important one is that fee-for-service medicine provides a strong incentive to overprovide services. But this also stems from consumers not being able to make effective decisions about the appropriate types and amounts of services they receive.

23. For more information on patient cost-sharing outside of the United States, see Section 4.3.2.

Figure 3.6 The Effect of Coinsurance on Welfare Loss

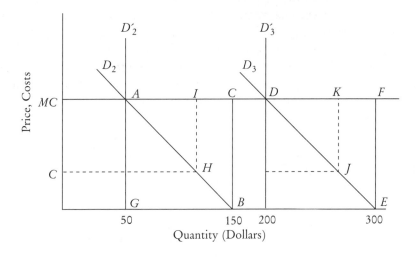

copayments, which in turn reduces utilization. Although this conclusion might seem surprising, it follows directly if one holds the viewpoint that the demand curve provides our best estimate of the benefits derived from the use of additional services.

U.S. health economists, more so than those from other countries, seem to be inclined to believe that patient cost-sharing should be encouraged as a primary means of achieving efficiency in the health area. Some of the most notable advocates of such a position were the researchers who conducted the RAND Health Insurance Experiment. One question these researchers asked was whether the experiment could justify its costs, which would exceed $200 million in today's dollars. They concluded that the experiment more than paid for itself because of its reduction in services that appeared to do little to improve health status:

> [W]e believe that the benefits of this particular experiment greatly exceeded the costs. . . . Between 1982 and 1984, there was a remarkable increase in initial cost sharing in the United States, at least for hospital services. For example, the number of major companies with first-dollar charges for hospital care rose from 30 to 63 percent in those two years, and the number of such firms with an annual deductible of $200 per person or more rose from 4 to 21 percent. Although it is impossible to know how much of this change can be attributed to the experimental results, the initial findings of the experiment were published . . . and given wide publicity in both the general and trade press. In certain instances a direct link between changes in cost sharing and the experimental results can be made. (Manning et al. 1987, 272)

Because the experiment showed that increased patient cost-sharing reduced medical expenditures, the researchers estimated that, under the most optimistic scenario, the eight-year experiment could have paid for itself in a week!

Non-U.S. health economists have been more amenable to the idea that a fee-for-service system could be efficient in the absence of patient cost-sharing. Robert Evans and colleagues argue that the case for patient cost-sharing is difficult to make if four questions can be answered in the affirmative:

- Is the service really health care?
- Does the service work?
- Is the service medically necessary?
- Is there no better alternative?

If a service passes all of these tests, "the standard argument against user charges, that they tax the sick, seems wholly justified" (Evans et al. 1983).

Currently there is a great deal of policy interest in the United States in medical savings accounts (MSAs), which rely heavily on patient cost-sharing. Under most MSA proposals, people (usually employees) would be able to choose a health plan with a very large annual deductible (often several thousand dollars), but which covers medical expenses above that amount in full. The savings in premiums could be used to make payments toward the deductible, or alternatively, to spend (or save) on anything that the consumer desires.

Here we will focus on three criticisms of MSAs that derive from the above discussion. First, it is not clear that MSAs will indeed quell the demand for services. Although it is likely that people with MSAs will forgo some minor services, the vast majority of medical spending goes toward "big ticket items." Two percent of the U.S. population in a particular year, for example, is responsible for over 40 percent of expenditures (Berk and Monheit 1992). Because any hospitalization or procedure is likely to meet the annual deductible, patients will not have much of a financial incentive to curb medical spending. For that reason, there is also little reason to expect that MSAs would result in depressed demand for expensive medical technologies.

Second, the idea behind MSAs is that individuals can make informed choices about whether treatment should be sought for a particular illness. It was shown earlier, however, that there is evidence that makes one doubt consumers' ability to perform this task very well.[24] Findings from

---

24. There is also concern whether consumers will make rational choices with regard to contributions to programs such as MSAs. In a study of university employees' contributions to tax-deductible

the RAND Health Insurance Study indicate that patients are as likely to forgo effective medical services in the presence of cost-sharing as they are to forgo less effective care (Lohr et al. 1986; Siu et al. 1986).

Third, selection bias could cause various problems for a country embarking on MSAs. One would expect those who are less likely to need medical care to be the most likely to purchase the accounts. This would cause two problems. First, patients who are sicker—and who therefore might need more incentive to consider costs when making medical care decisions—would not tend to enroll in MSAs, and therefore would not be subject to any efficiency-enhancing incentives that derive from cost-sharing. Second, it would mean that the markets would be segmented, with healthier people in these less expensive plans and sicker people pooled together in non-MSA plans, making them even more expensive.

Two broad arguments can be made against employing patient cost-sharing as a cost-control technique. First, of course, is the issue of equity. It is frequently argued that cost-sharing is more burdensome on people with lower incomes. In this regard, one of the key findings of the RAND study was that the health of the sick and the poor was most adversely affected by cost-sharing (Newhouse et al. 1993).[25]

The other issue concerns efficiency—specifically, are there alternative ways of encouraging efficiency and containing health costs besides cost-sharing? Two U.S. health economists mentioned earlier, Ellis and McGuire (1993), have argued the benefits of what they deem to be a "neglected" area of reform, supply-side cost-sharing, "which seeks to alter the incentives of health care workers to provide certain services" (p. 135). (One could make a compelling argument that this has not been neglected by analysts in other countries, however.) With supply-side policies, Ellis and McGuire argue, it is possible to reach the same desired level of quantity as with demand-side levers. Furthermore, they claim that supply-side cost-sharing is clearly superior to traditional demand-side policies in one key respect: it does not result in a financial burden on patients.

Nevertheless, economists tend to focus most of their attention on the role of price. One possible reason, noted by Milton Friedman, was given

---

flexible spending accounts, Schweitzer, Hershey, and Asch (1996) found that employees did not act rationally. Relatively few contributed to such accounts, even though it would have been in the best interest financially of most to have done so. And those who did contribute tended to give the same dollar contribution each year, even when their changing financial circumstances would have been expected to result in different contribution levels amounts over time. The authors conclude that "[t]he pervasiveness of these patterns raises concerns that health care reform plans that rely on financial incentives at the consumer level—for example, proposed medical savings accounts—will be inefficient (p. 583).

25. For a summary of literature on the effect of cost-sharing, see Rice and Morrison (1994).

in Section 2.2: it is part of an overall division of labor between economics and the other social sciences. If each of the social sciences were equally influential in influencing policy, this would not present a problem. But a strong case can be made that economics seems to be paramount among the social sciences in its influence over health policy. Given that, it is incumbent on health economists to consider other health policy levers as well.

Although one could imagine many possible policy levers—and indeed, several supply-side levers will be discussed in Section 4.3—the focus here will be on a single, nonprice demand-side lever—influencing behavior. It is curious that many economists, who are concerned about the purported welfare loss due to excess health insurance, do not focus on more tangible losses—such as the cost of "bad" behaviors from things like smoking, alcohol consumption, drug abuse, and so forth. This is not to say that health economists do not study such issues—they do—but rather that these costs are often not viewed as welfare losses for society. This is particularly curious given the estimated sizes of these losses: in the United States alone, an estimated $67 billion annually for drug abuse, $99 billion for alcohol abuse, and $91 billion for smoking (Robert Wood Johnson Foundation 1994). These figures far exceed all estimates of the welfare losses from health insurance.

Sociologists and psychologists have been concerned about the factors that influence behavior, and ways in which it can be altered. The field of health education focuses, to a large degree, on how behaviors can be changed. Mechanic (1979) has stated that

> [r]educing needs involves the prevention of illness or diminishing patients' psychological dependence on the medical encounter for social support or other secondary advantages. Reducing desire for services requires changing people's views of the value of different types of medical care, making them more aware of the real costs of service in relation to the benefits received, and legitimizing alternatives for dealing with many problems. (p. 11)

The task of changing behavior is not easy, however. In this regard, he writes, "[I]t is prudent to recognize the difficulty of the task, the forces working against change, and the depths of ignorance concerning the origins of these behaviors and the ways in which they can best be modified" (p. 12).

The point is not that economists need to be conducting this research. Rather, it is that (1) policy levers like these need to be recognized by health economists who are proposing policy; and (2) relying on conventional tools such as demand elasticities to recommend policy is inappropriate once some of the special characteristics of the health market are recognized.

3.3.3 Should People Pay More for Price-Elastic Services?

Another generally accepted tool in the health economist's toolbox is that the magnitude of patient coinsurance rates should be directly related to the elasticity of demand. More specifically, services for which consumers show a high demand elasticity should have higher cost-sharing requirements than services for which consumers are less price sensitive. As we shall see, the basis for this argument is similar to the one used by economists in arguing that there is a welfare loss associated with excessive amounts of health insurance.

Ellis and McGuire (1993) summarize the issue as follows:

> [T]he optimal insurance literature has been based on the assumption that the demand curve correctly reflects the marginal benefits of services. As a result, it has held that the greater the demand response to what consumer/patients must pay for health care, the higher should be demand-side cost sharing. (p. 137)

Why is this the case? Suppose one views the demand curve as indicating the marginal benefits a consumer derives from a service. In Figure 3.7, point P_1 shows the price of medical care in the absence of health insurance, and point P_2, the price when a person has insurance that pays 80 percent of medical costs. Thus, at point C, which represents the quantity of medical care purchased with insurance, the marginal benefits derived from the last service are only one-fifth as great as at point A, where the person is uninsured.

As noted earlier, under the conventional theory this results in a societal welfare loss, which is equal to the difference between the costs of producing the last service Q_2—indicated by point B—and the benefits as shown at point C. But that is the welfare loss associated with only the last service. There is also welfare loss for all other services purchased between Q_1 and Q_2. The total welfare loss is therefore equal to the triangle ABC.[26]

Now suppose that the demand curve is steeper, or less elastic (curve D'). In the figure, when the person obtains insurance, thereby lowering the price of care, he or she increases his consumption only to Q'. In this case, it is clear that the welfare loss will be smaller, equaling the triangle AEF rather than ABC. Similarly, one can imagine that if the demand curve is more gently sloped (that is, more price elastic), health insurance will result in a larger welfare-loss triangle.

---

26. As noted earlier, one needs to weigh this welfare loss in the conventional theory against the welfare gain from the reduction in risk brought about by the insurance. For convenience, we do not consider the latter element here, but this does not affect the substance of the argument.

Figure 3.7   Relationship Between Demand Elasticity and Welfare Loss

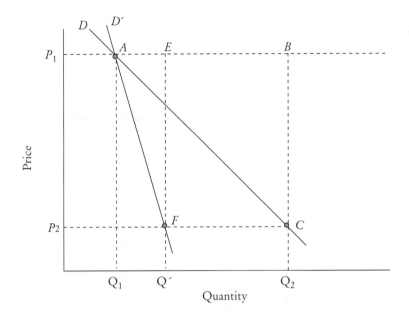

The intuition behind this result is straightforward. If the possession of insurance leads to a large increase in utilization, then welfare loss will be larger because more services will be purchased where the marginal costs exceed marginal benefits. Thus, one would improve social welfare by assessing higher patient coinsurance rates for such services, thereby reducing usage. In contrast, if utilization rates are not very sensitive to the possession of insurance, then there is little welfare loss, and less need to charge high coinsurance rates.

It should now be clear that conventional theory calls for higher coinsurance rates when services are more responsive to out-of-pocket price. We therefore need to consider what services are the most price elastic, since those are the ones that the theory tells us should have the highest patient cost-sharing requirements.

The major source of data to answer this question is the RAND Health Insurance Experiment. Its results in this regard are somewhat ambiguous because the calculated elasticities vary depending on the level of coinsurance. In the study, patients were assessed 0 percent or 25 percent or 95 percent of the total charge.[27] Therefore, to examine

---

27. Some patients were charged 50 percent coinsurance rates, but they were not used in the analysis of demand elasticities.

Table 3.3 Arc Price Elasticities of Medical Spending in the RAND Health Insurance Experiment

Patient Share of Charges	Acute Care Services	Chronic Care Services	Well-Care Services	Total Outpatient Services	Hospital Services	Total Medical Services	Dental Care Services
0%–25%	−0.16	−0.20	−0.14	−0.17	−0.17	−0.17	−0.12
25%–95%	−0.32	−0.23	−0.43	−0.31	−0.14	−0.22	−0.39

Source: Newhouse, J. P., et al. 1993. *Free for All?: Lessons from the RAND Health Insurance Experiment* (Harvard University Press, Cambridge, MA), p. 121.

price responsiveness to alternative coinsurance rates, one can do so only between these intervals.

These elasticities are shown in Table 3.3. In general, the elasticities do not vary a great deal by type of service. One noteworthy exception is that so-called "well-care services," which, while showing a comparable elasticity to other outpatient services (acute and chronic) in the 0 percent to 25 percent range, had a much larger one in the 25 percent to 95 percent range (Phelps 1992, 123). Dental services also showed a relatively high elasticity in the 25 percent to 95 percent rage. The well-care services considered in the study would include preventive care, but other services as well.

The implications of the standard economic model are nevertheless clear: if preventive services are the most price responsive, they should have the highest patient coinsurance rates, which in turn will discourage their usage. This would be true even if it were shown that some of these services were particularly effective in improving health and/or well-being.

There are, of course, alternative criteria that one could use in determining patient copayment levels that are in the best interest of society. One model, popular in a number of recent proposals for U.S. health reform, would have made preventive services free of any copayments— the *opposite* of what the economic model would recommend.

There are several possible justifications for basing copayment rates on factors other than price elasticities, all of which have been discussed above in other contexts. First is the issue of whether consumers have sufficient information. If they do not, then they are likely to underestimate the value of investing in preventive services. Second, even if the appropriate information is available, people may not use it correctly. As noted, it is difficult for people to make choices based on counterfactual information. Furthermore, because of people's tendency toward cognitive dissonance, they may avoid seeking some types of services that are of value to them.

Third, medical experts may be better aware of the benefits of certain services than are individuals—and these experts routinely recommend more services than people are obtaining. Fourth, people might be short-sighted in their views, particularly when they are young. Finally, there is a public good aspect of preventive care. If it makes you healthy I want you to have it, but the free-rider effect (discussed in Chapter 2) will prevent me from subsidizing you. Subsidized, low copayments for preventive care therefore could meet this demand.

The point is that, when one assumes that a demand curve for medical services represents the marginal benefits consumers receive from services, then certain policy implications follow. One such implication is that patients should be charged more for services that are price sensitive. But if one does not make such strong assumptions about the meaning of demand curves for health services, then a different set of policy prescriptions would seem to be more appropriate. One example is reducing patient prices for preventive services even if such services are more price responsive than others—a conclusion directly in conflict with that provided by conventional theory.

3.3.4 Can People Choose the Right Health Plan?

A successful competitive market depends on information: the availability of good information about alternative choices, as well as the ability of consumers to make proper use of this information. The success of most market-based approaches to reform relies on people choosing the right health plan—one that delivers high-quality services in a cost-effective manner. To accomplish this, people need to have and use information about alternative plan choices.

Researchers, however, know very little about how well consumers could discern plan quality from the written materials that would be distributed through health plan report cards. Even if the information were collected by an independent organization—which is *not* the case currently—there is no evidence to indicate that consumers would be able to use such information effectively. As discussed earlier, researchers have found that consumers do not understand much of what is included on report cards, ignoring much of the "objective" information provided (such as utilization rates for preventive services), and overinterpreting other measures that they find more intuitive, such as simple satisfaction (Hibbard and Jewett 1997).

Relevant here is a study Judith Hibbard and Jacqueline Jewett (1996) conducted on the type of information consumers look for on report cards. The authors found that most consumers indicate that the key types of information for them in choosing a health plan are so-called "desirable events" such as utilization rates for mammograms, cholesterol screening, and pediatric immunizations. Less important to them are "undesirable events" such as hospital death rates from heart attacks, rates of low birth weights, and hospital-acquired infections. Curiously, then, when given report cards on two alterative health plans—one with a better record on desirable events and the other with a better record on undesirable events—consumers overwhelmingly chose the latter. Although far more research is needed in this area, this evidence casts doubt on how well consumers can use report card information to make the best choices for themselves. The mere existence and dissemination of information, even if objective and complete, does not guarantee that an individual will use it properly.

Finally, under competitive-based reform proposals, there is an intense pressure on the part of health plans to attract enrollees by keeping premiums at a competitive level. One way to do this is through enacting true efficiencies, but another is to try to obtain a *favorable selection* of patients. It is in the interest of plans to avoid groups whose costs are likely to be high, and individuals with chronic conditions (Light 1995).[28] In addition, because enrolling in better health plans is likely to be more expensive, it is possible that the lowest-cost plans in an area will be the least desirable ones—for example, the ones having a limited provider network, offering little choice, paying for only the most basic services, making it difficult to obtain referrals, and so forth (Rice, Brown, and Wyn 1993). Indeed, to the extent that putting providers at considerable risk is effective in controlling costs, one would expect less expensive plans to employ more severe physician incentives to conserve resources.

---

28. One way to deal with this problem would be to "risk-adjust" payments to health plans— that is, to pay them more if they have sicker patients. Although health services researchers are devoting much attention to this problem, there are few instances in which health plan contributions use risk adjustment, and in most of those cases, adjustments are done based just on demographic characteristics of enrollees, such as age and sex.

4

SUPPLY THEORY

BESIDES DEMAND, the other key element in understanding microeconomics is supply theory. Supply is usually defined as the amount of goods and services firms wish to sell at alternative prices. In a competitive market, the point at which demand and supply are equal indicates both the price at which goods and services will be exchanged, and the amount exchanged.

In most economic applications, supply plays a subsidiary role to demand. In general, if demand for a product changes because, say, people's tastes change, firms will produce less; similarly, if people demand more of a good, firms will tend to increase production and/or more firms will enter the market in order to meet this additional demand.

The health services market is different from others in this respect, however: supply considerations play a very important role in determining both prices and output. This is true primarily because suppliers are not just passive producers of whatever is demanded. Rather, as in the case of the physician, who acts as the patient's agent, suppliers can play a major role in determining what services the consumer ultimately chooses to purchase. Because of this, the list of policy tools available in the health sector is much more extensive than in most other aspects of the economy.

Section 4.1 briefly summarizes traditional supply theory; readers already familiar with the derivation and determinants of supply can skip this material. Section 4.2 provides a critique of supply theory based largely on doubts about the validity of the assumptions presented earlier. Section 4.3 then discusses several applications of this critique to the area of health policy.

4.1 The Traditional Economic Model

Section 2.1.2 provided a brief summary of production theory. It showed how firms are expected to choose both the level of inputs and the level of outputs to maximize profits. Here, we modify Figure 2.5 to indicate how a firm's supply curve is constructed; this is shown in Figure 4.1. As before, *MC* shows the marginal cost of production and *P* is the market price. The curve *AVC* is *average variable costs* of production; curve *ATC* shows *average total costs*.

To understand these curves, one needs to know that total costs are subdivided into variable and fixed costs. Variable costs are those that change as the level of output changes, whereas fixed costs are those—such as capital purchases and land—that do not. The *ATC* curve shows the average total costs of producing each level of quantity, whereas *AVC* shows the average of all costs except for fixed costs.[1] The reason the curves gravitate toward each other as quantity increases is because the

Figure 4.1   Economic Profits and Supply

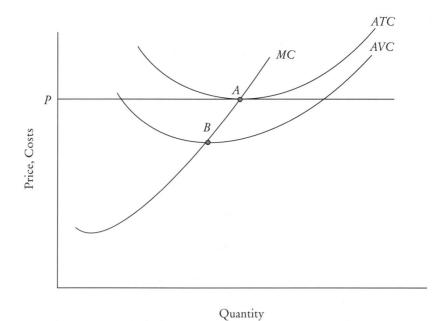

---

1. These curves are drawn such that *MC* intersects both *AVC* and *ATC* at their minimum points. There is a mathematical certainty. When *MC*—the cost of the last unit—is higher than average costs *AVC* or *ATC*, it brings the average up. In contrast, when the last unit is less costly than the average, it brings the average down. Thus, the only point at which *MC* can be equal to *AVC* and *ATC* is at their minimum, where these curves are neither rising nor falling.

difference between the two—*average fixed costs*—declines as quantity rises.[2]

At point *A*, the firm neither makes any economic profits nor suffers any economic losses because the price received for selling each unit of output is exactly equal to *ATC*. This lack of profits is not a concern to the economist, however, because the economic definition of costs includes an item for a "normal" rate of return on investment. Zero economic profits simply means that the firm is making a profit equal to the typical rate of return available on other investments. In a competitive market, firms are expected to have an economic profit rate of zero.[3]

Recall that to maximize profits, a firm produces at the point where the marginal cost of production equals the market price. As can be seen from Figure 4.1, all points on the *MC* curves that are below and to the left of point *A* are money losers, because at any corresponding level of quantity, *ATC* exceeds price. Note that between points *A* and *B*, the firm will lose money, but the market price still exceeds the firm's average variable costs. Thus, at least in the short run, the firm would be willing to stay in business because proceeds cover expenses. Below and to the left of point *B*, however, the market price does not even cover these variable costs. Unless the firm has some reason to believe that things will be different in the future, the sensible decision is to shut down.

The portion of the *MC* curve above point *B* is defined as the short-run *supply curve* for a competitive firm. All points on this curve show how much a profit-maximizing firm would be willing to produce at different price levels. This can be seen simply by drawing several horizontal lines, indicating alternative market prices, that intersect *MC*. Each of the intersections represents a profit-maximizing level of output; the set of all such points above and to the right of point *B* is therefore the firm's supply curve. *Aggregate* supply—how much is supplied by the combination of all firms in a market—is simply the sum of each firm's individual supply.

We will not deal with the concept of the long-run supply curve here because it is does not provide insights used later in the chapter. Briefly, in the long run, all costs are variable; the firm must choose not only the right level of variable inputs, but also its scale of operation (e.g., capital stock) in order to maximize profits.

---

2. Average fixed costs are defined as total fixed costs (*FC*) divided by quantity produced (*Q*). By definition, *FC*, the numerator, does not change as output increases, but quantity, the denominator, obviously does. Thus, as quantity rises average fixed costs decline, which means that *AVC* and *ATC* will converge.

3. This is because at positive profit levels, more firms will enter the market and/or existing firms will produce more, thereby raising market supply and depressing market prices until equilibrium is reached at the zero-profit level.

A supply curve shows the relationship between different levels of market price and the amount of a good or service supplied by a firm. Its upward-sloping shape indicates that the firm would wish to supply more when the market price is higher and less when the market price is lower. Higher prices would result in more profits, and therefore an incentive to produce more. Lower prices, however, would result in lower profits. In order to maximize profits, the firm would cut back on its last, most costly units of production.[4]

There are several factors that can cause a supply curve to shift. Two notable ones are the prices of inputs and technology.[5] We can therefore write the firm's supply schedule as:

$$S = f(P, P_i, T), \qquad (4.1)$$

where S is the amount of the good supplied, P is its market price, P_i is the price of inputs, and T is the level of technology.

Suppose that a technological breakthrough reduces the cost of production. This would mean that, at any price, the firm could profitably produce more; or alternatively, at any quantity, the costs of production would be lower. This means that the *supply curve* (examples of which are shown later in the chapter, in Figure 4.2) would shift outward. If the cost of inputs declines, the firm's supply curve would shift for the same reason. It is notable that most analysts in the health area find technology to be, on average, cost increasing rather than cost decreasing.[6] If this is true, it is probably because the technologies being used are designed not to reduce cost so much as to improve people's health status and/or comfort.

The exact relationship between the quantity of a good supplied and its price is called the *elasticity of supply*. It is defined as the percentage change in the quantity of a good supplied, divided by the percentage change in its price. A supply elasticity of +0.3 means that when the market price rises by, say, 10 percent, the quantity supplied increases by 3 percent.

The above model of supply depends on a number of assumptions. The validity of those assumptions that play an important role in health policy are assessed in the following section.

---

4. See Chapter 2, footnote 5, for a discussion of why marginal costs are expected to rise as quantity increases.

5. Other factors sometimes listed in textbooks include expectations about the future market price level, taxes, and the prices of related goods produced by the firm.

6. For a good discussion of these issues, see Newhouse (1993). Another example is that each year, the Health Care Financing Administration divides the annual increase in national health expenditures into four categories: population, economywide inflation, health inflation, and "other factors." This last category is usually about one-third of the total cause of inflation, and represents growth in the quantity and intensity of services, much of which is a result of technological growth.

4.2 Problems with the Traditional Model

In the traditional economic model, demand is key; supply is essentially along for the ride. Of course, to obtain the market price and quantity, one needs both. Beyond that, however, the role of supply is rather passive. If, for example, demand shifts outward, causing a short-run increase in prices, quantities, and profits, supply will increase to meet this demand. In contrast, a change in supply—perhaps due to a reduction in the cost of obtaining inputs—does not influence people's demand curve, which is a function primarily of tastes (or, in the health area, health status).

If policymakers wish to alter a *competitive* market for some reason, traditional economic theory would suggest focusing on demand. There are only a few limited tools available for doing so, however. The main one, of course, is price. Taxes can be used to raise prices, thus suppressing the amount of a good that is demanded, and subsidies can do the opposite. A second policy lever might be to improve consumers' information so that they can make choices that are in their best interest. Beyond that, the list of demand-side tools is rather thin.

If, however, suppliers are not merely passive actors in the operation of the market, the list of policy tools available is considerably expanded. Among the most prominent set of these in the health area are incentives designed to influence providers' behavior. Capitation, DRGs, and practice guidelines represent a few such examples. Thus, to determine which set of policy tools are most appropriate, in this section we examine the extent to which the assumptions of the competitive model in the area of supply are or are not met in the health sector. The policy implications of this analysis are then provided in Section 4.3.

In this section, we critique five assumptions of the competitive model, which were presented in Chapter 1:

Assumption 10. Supply and demand are independently determined.

Assumption 11. Firms do not have any monopoly power.

Assumption 12. Firms maximize profits.

Assumption 13. There are not increasing returns to scale.

Assumption 14. Production is independent of the distribution of wealth.

4.2.1 Are Supply and Demand Independently Determined?

This issue, oddly enough, is one of the most studied in all of health economics; but it is also one in which there seems to be the least agreement. Most of the focus has been on whether suppliers—particularly physicians—act totally in their patients' interest, or if alternatively, they can succeed in convincing their patients to act in a way that also benefits them (the suppliers). In the literature, this has been couched in terms of whether physicians act as perfect *agents* for their patients, or even more commonly, in terms of whether physicians can *induce demand* among patients for their services.

One reason that demand inducement has engendered so much interest among health economists is that its existence is so totally at odds with the competitive model. Normally, we would expect that an increase in supply would lower price, but that is not necessarily the case if physicians induce demand. Furthermore, we would also expect physicians to supply fewer services if they are paid less per service, but again, this would not necessarily be true if demand inducement were present.[7]

As noted, there is little agreement on the issue, although most health economists seem to believe that physicians are able to induce demand to some extent. In a survey of almost 300 U.S. and Canadian health economists, Roger Feldman and Michael Morrisey (1990) report that 81 percent of respondents believe that physicians generate demand for their own services. But many economists seem to have considerable doubt concerning physicians' ability to hoodwink patients into demanding far more services than they really want. Perhaps a good summary of the state of the art is provided by Jeremiah Hurley and Roberta Labelle (1995), who conclude,

> It appears that, in response to economic considerations . . . physicians *can* induce demand for their services, they *sometimes do* induce demand, but that such responses are neither automatic nor unconstrained. Further, physicians do not always respond in ways that can be predicted. (p. 420)

This section is not intended to definitively answer any of the questions that surround demand inducement. Rather, it tries to show that in spite of the difficulty of testing for demand inducement, there is enough available evidence to make one doubt the independence of demand and supply curves in the physicians' services market. Readers wishing to examine both sides of the issue may wish to consult a published debate.[8]

This section is divided into four parts, the first three of which are devoted to different ways of testing for demand inducement, and the last of which provides some summary remarks.

---

7. One possible exception to this is if physicians have a "backward-bending" labor supply curve, which is discussed below.

8. For the anti-inducement side, see Feldman and Sloan (1988). For a contrasting opinion, see Rice and Labelle (1989).

Testing Demand Inducement Through Physician-Population Ratios

One of the earliest methods of testing whether physicians induce demand was to determine how some market measure, such as utilization or price, changes in response to a change in the number of physicians. The idea behind the test is straightforward: if there is an increase in competition among physicians and physicians can induce demand, they will do so to maintain their revenues. Many such studies have been conducted, some of which find evidence of demand inducement and others of which do not.[9] Due to inherent difficulties in conducting such studies, however, it is unlikely that they will ever reveal uncontestable evidence.

Some of the problems can be seen from Figure 4.2, which is taken from earlier articles by Uwe Reinhardt (1978) and by the author (Rice 1983).[10] D_0 and S_0 are the initial demand and supply curves, and S_1 reflects an independent or exogenous increase in the physician-population ratio. D_1 is the demand curve if physicians induce demand in response to the increase in competition. Clearly, just looking at whether utilization increases in response to more physicians does not distinguish between the competitive and demand-inducement hypotheses—both predict utilization to increase (from Q_0 to Q_c with no inducement, and from Q_0 to Q_i with inducement). But the problem goes beyond even that. Suppose that equilibrium price and quantity move from point A to point C. Although this would seem to be consistent with the inducement model, note that it would also be consistent with a no-inducement scenario if the initial demand curve were D' rather than D_0, as shown by the dotted line. Since it is very difficult to obtain data that tell us the exact shape of demand curves, it seems even less likely that examining changes in utilization can help us determine whether physicians induce demand in response to changes in the number of physicians in an area.

Another possibility is to look at what happens to price as evidence about demand inducement. But, as drawn, both models predict a decline in price. If physicians do not induce demand, market price will decline from P_0 to P_c, and if they do induce demand, from P_0 to P_i. This may seem a bit artificial, however, because one can imagine D_1 drawn in such a

9. A few notable studies that find evidence of inducement using physician-population ratios include Evans, Parish, and Sully (1973); Fuchs (1978); Hemenway and Fallon (1985); Cromwell and Mitchell (1986); and Tussing and Wojtowycz (1986). Some studies concluding that demand inducement is not terribly significant include Wilensky and Rossiter (1983); McCarthy (1985); Stano (1985); and Escarce (1992).

10. Reinhardt's article also shows that two other ways of examining inducement—output per physician and income per physician—also provide ambiguous results.

Figure 4.2 Effect of an Increase in the Number of Physicians in a
Geographic Area

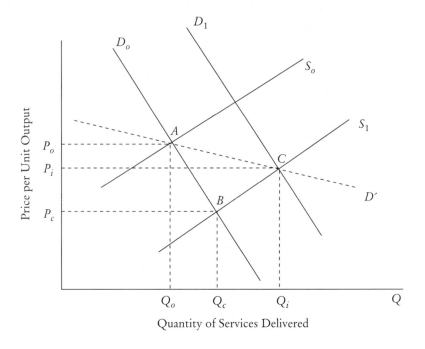

Source: Rice, T. H. 1983, "The Impact of Changing Medicare Reimbursement Rates on Physician-Induced Demand," *Medical Care* 21 (8): 805.

way that price would actually rise above P_o. Nevertheless, it would seem
that one way to determine whether physicians induce demand is to see
if price *rises* in response to an increase in the number of physicians. If it
does, then it would seem that physicians are inducing demand, although
a decline in price, as just demonstrated, would not provide evidence one
way or the other.

Unfortunately, there are also problems with this method. The primary one is a statistical issue known as *omitted variables bias*. Suppose that
we do indeed find that areas with more physicians have higher prices. This
would seem to be consistent with the demand-inducement hypothesis,
but only if we adequately control for all of the other factors that would
make one area of the country more expensive than others. It might be
that physicians gravitate to attractive urban and suburban settings with
various cultural amenities, good schools, and the like—areas that tend to
have higher price levels. If data are not available to capture all of these

subtle yet important characteristics of an area, then we might incorrectly attribute higher physician prices to demand inducement.

Finally, Joseph Newhouse (1978) points out another problem with drawing conclusions about demand inducement by looking at the relationship between market price and physician supply:

> Recall that analysis of a competitive market assumes a fixed and homogeneous product. But physicians in areas with greater concentration of physicians spend more time with their patients and patients in such areas spend less time waiting for their physicians. More time with the physician and less waiting time are both desirable characteristics that lead to more physician time per visit. In a competitive market, visits using more physician time would be more expensive. As a result, even if the market were competitive, there could be a positive relationship between the physician/population ratio and the price of a (non-homogenous) physician visit. The test of demand creation based on physician prices also fails. (p. 60)

Testing Demand Inducement Through Physician Payment Rates

Perhaps a somewhat more promising method of testing for demand inducement is to determine how physicians respond to changes in the payments they receive. In general, one might expect that, without demand inducement, physicians would provide fewer services when they face a decline in payment—they would simply slide down the supply curve. But with demand inducement, they might behave differently—say, increasing the provision of services in the wake of payment reductions in order to recoup lost income. Note that this sort of behavior is *not* consistent with the upward-sloping supply curve that is typically assumed in competitive markets.

Most, but certainly not all, of the evidence on demand inducement using these methods supports its existence.[11] In one of the earliest sets of studies, researchers from the Urban Institute found that California physicians increased the quantity and intensity of services provided to Medicare beneficiaries in response to a freeze in program payment rates during the early 1970s (Holahan and Scanlon 1979; Hadley, Holahan, and Scanlon 1979). In another set of studies, the present author found that physicians in urban areas of Colorado, who faced declines in their Medicare payment rates during the late 1970s compared to their nonurban colleagues, increased the intensity of medical and surgical services, and the amount of surgery provided and laboratory tests ordered (Rice 1983;

---

11. A review of much of the earlier literature (through the early 1980s) can be found in Gabel and Rice (1985).

Rice 1984). Other researchers have found that physicians responded to Medicare payment rate freezes during the mid-1980s by increasing the quantity and/or intensity of surgery, radiology, and special diagnostic tests (Mitchell, Wedig, and Cromwell 1989).

Finally, a study of the Canadian experience through the early 1980s showed that provinces that were least generous in raising physician payment rates over time experienced the greatest increase in the volume and intensity of services provided (Barer, Evans, and Labelle 1988). Unlike most other studies, this one could not be criticized for ignoring changes in patient out-of-pocket costs because during this period Canadians received services without any copayments. In contrast, one confounding factor in most U.S. studies is that reduced physician payment rates often result in lower patient copayments (e.g., the patient pays 20 percent of charges, which have declined). Thus, if the physician provides more services after the payment reduction, it is possible that part of the reason is that patient demand increased as a result of lower copayments.

There has been some counterevidence, however. A study using data from some of the Canadian provinces found little relationship over a dozen years between utilization of specific procedures and their fees (Hurley, Labelle, and Rice 1990). Some studies of Medicare payment rate reductions for so-called "overvalued procedures" (mainly surgery and testing) in the late 1980s found little evidence that physicians increased the quantity of services provided (Escarce 1993a, 1993b). Other studies of the same payment reductions do find evidence of volume increases in the wake of Medicare payment reductions, (Physician Payment Review Commission 1993).

There is one problem with all of this literature, that Hurley and Labelle (1995) point out. As in the case with testing demand inducement with physician-population ratios, results derived by examining response to physician payment rate changes may be consistent both with a demand inducement and with a competitive model of physician behavior (Hurley and Labelle 1995). Suppose that physicians have a normal, upward-sloping supply curve. If payment rates decrease, we would therefore expect the volume of services supplied to decrease. Consequently, if there is an increase in the amount of services provided in response to a payment reduction, then this would provide evidence of demand inducement (assuming any alternative explanations can be invalidated).

This conclusion is based on the assumption that physicians attempt to maximize their income (see Section 4.2.3, below). Most evidence indicates that this is not the case, however. Things that also matter to physicians include, perhaps most importantly, the availability of leisure time. Other commonly noted elements of a physician's utility function

Figure 4.3 Backward-Bending Supply Curve

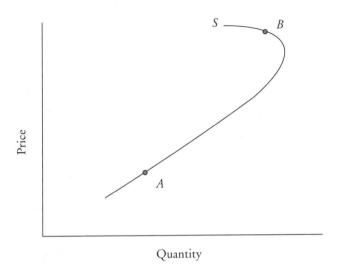

are professional ethics (e.g., having the patient's interest at heart or alternatively, distaste toward inducing services) and having an interesting caseload.

If a physician tries to maximize both income and leisure jointly, it is possible that his or her supply curve will exhibit a "backward-bending" shape. At low levels of fees—for example, point *A* in Figure 4.3— higher payment rates will induce more work. At some level, such as point *B*, unit payment rates are so high that the physician may decide to enjoy more leisure as fees climb even higher. Thus, a reduction in payment rates would lead to an *increase* in the quantity supplied. Note that this is the same result as under demand inducement—but without there being any inducement whatsoever. As Hurley and Labelle (1995) note, "[O]ne cannot empirically distinguish the inducement and no-inducement models based on predicted utilization effects" (p. 424).

Other Methods of Testing Demand Inducement[12]

Partly as a result of the difficulty in using the above strategies for analyzing demand inducement, some analysts have employed other means. One novel approach has been to see whether physicians and their families use more or fewer medical services than other people, the theory being that if physicians induce demand among their patients, they and their families are likely to avail themselves to fewer (unnecessary) services than others.

---

12. For a thorough list of different approaches, see Labelle, Stoddart, and Rice (1994).

Two studies that have examined this have found, however, that physicians and their families use *more* services than others, thus contradicting the notion of demand inducement (Bunker and Brown 1974; Hay and Leahy 1982).[13] One problem with studies like these, however, is the difficulty of controlling for the fact that physicians, other medical providers, and their families often get care at much cheaper prices. In addition, it is hard to account for other differences between medically oriented and other families.[14]

A final approach is to ask physicians how much money they would like to make and compare this to their actual income. Then it is possible to determine whether this differential is correlated with their practice behavior. In one such study, it was found that the farther physicians were below their targeted income, the more they charged their patients—evidence of demand inducement (Rizzo and Blumenthal 1996).[15]

Summary Remarks

It should now be sufficiently clear that there likely will always be doubts about how much demand physicians induce among their patients. Part of this is due to the inherent ambiguity in the tools available, as the above discussion implies. We simply do not have sufficient information available to answer the question definitively. Gavin Mooney (1994) has stated that, to understand whether patients are being *induced* to use more services than they really want, we need to know how many they would demand if they were as well informed as the physician, but no such studies have ever been conducted. Reinhardt (1989) makes a similar point when he states,

> [H]ighly sophisticated econometric methods ultimately cannot define what proportion of observed utilization [is] simply *accepted* by sick patients (or their anxious relatives) and what proportion the latter would have *demanded* of their own free will, had they been as well informed as their physicians. (p. 339)

There may be another, very different reason why agreement is likely never to be reached, however. It is because the issue of demand inducement seems to raise the hackles of followers of conventional economic theory. Reinhardt (1985) makes this point, writing that

---

13. The Bunker and Brown study was not about demand inducement per se, because it was written before the debate started to rage.

14. One possible difference is that health professionals are less tolerant than others of uncertainty with regard to their own health, and therefore demand more services when they are patients in an effort to minimize this uncertainty (Harold Luft, personal communication).

15. For critiques of this research, see the Commentaries by Thomas McGuire and Uwe Reinhardt, along with the authors' reply, in the same issue of the journal.

[o]ne suspects that vested interest in neoclassical economic theory has added at least some fuel to the flames. Mastery of the neoclassical framework requires a heavy personal investment on the part of the analyst. Among the payoffs to that investment is entree into a fraternity whose power has derived in good part from the unity of thought forged by this shared analytic paradigm. One need not be an utter cynic to believe that, quite apart from our profession's yearning for truth, the defense of that unifying framework can take on a life of its own. (pp. 187–88)

Although there has been great disagreement over the subject, demand inducement is becoming less of a policy issue in the United States. In the early 1990s, the issue garnered some national attention when the Department of Health and Human Services (DHHS) drafted Medicare payment rates, under the new Medicare fee schedule, that were 16 percent lower than the medical profession had anticipated, in large part because of the *anticipation of* physician-induced demand in the wake of lower payment rates.[16] With the increased penetration of HMOs, demand inducement is not as pressing an issue. Even if physicians can induce demand, they do not have a financial incentive to do so when they are paid on a capitated or a salary basis. Nevertheless, the issue is relevant to discussions of the competitiveness of the marketplace for health services.

4.2.2 Do Firms Have Monopoly Power?

Of the 15 assumptions about a competitive market that are discussed in this book, this one has perhaps received the most attention from economists. Monopolies exist when only one firm sells a particular product in a market, but *monopoly power* means something a bit more subtle. A firm has monopoly power if it can raise prices without losing its entire market. When a firm has monopoly power, it can charge more than can a firm in a competitive market. And because conventional theory assumes that suppliers cannot influence demand, these higher prices will mean that the amount of output demanded will be lower than in a competitive market.

Figure 4.4 shows the conventional analysis of how monopolists and competitive firms compare with regard to pricing and output. To understand the drawing, one needs to know that monopolists maximize their profits by producing up to the point where the marginal revenue derived from providing an additional service equals the marginal cost of providing that service. They then set price at the highest level the market will bear, which is the point on the demand curve that corresponds to

---

16. After an outcry by the medical profession, DHHS dropped the assumption that physicians would respond to lower payment rates through demand inducement.

Figure 4.4 Pricing and Output Decisions by Competitive Firms and Monopolists

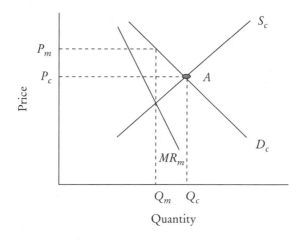

(i.e., is directly above) the profit-maximizing quantity of output. In the figure, S_c and D_c are the supply and demand curves in a competitive market, and MR_m is the monopolist's marginal revenue curve.[17] The output produced by competitive firms is indicated by point A, where the supply and demand curves intersect, as well as the corresponding output levels P_c and Q_c. The monopolist, however, produces less (Q_m) and charges more (P_m).

Because monopoly power has been studied so thoroughly, we will deal with it only briefly in this section. Clearly in the area of health services, firms have monopoly power. If a hospital raises its charges for a room, it possibly may lose some business, but obviously it will not lose all of its business. This is true for a number of reasons: hospitals differ with respect to quality, amenities, and location; patients may wish to be treated by a physician who prefers one hospital over another; and patients tend to pay out-of-pocket only a small fraction—about 3 percent—of the total hospital bill (Burner and Waldo 1995).

Similarly, as indicated in the previous section, physicians also appear to have some degree of monopoly power, as indicted by their ability to

---

17. If there is only one price at which all output is sold, the marginal revenue curve must be below the demand curve for a monopolist. This is because if the firm wishes to increase output by one unit, its marginal revenue increases by an amount less than the market price at which the output sells. This is true, in turn, because the firm must lower the price it receives on all of the goods sold, not just the last one. If, in contrast, a monopolist can charge a different price to all customers (or different classes of customers), then it can reap even higher profits. Such monopolists are called *price discriminators* due to their ability to charge different prices to different buyers.

Figure 4.5 Pricing and Output Decisions by Competitive Firms and Monopolists with Demand Inducement

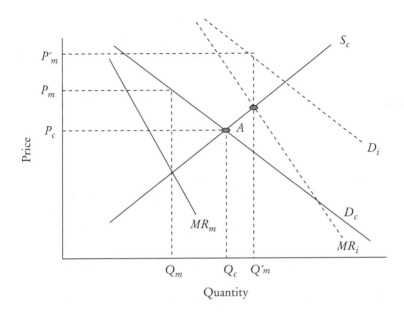

induce demand for their services, which in turn allows them to derive even greater profits. This is because suppliers can shift the demand and marginal revenue curves in Figure 4.5 to the slashed curves D_i and MR_i. This would result in the (monopolist) physician producing more than would be predicted by the conventional monopoly model (Q'_m), and charging more as well (P'_m).

In the United States, at the time of writing, there is a strong movement toward more monopoly power in two other key components of the health services market: hospitals and health plans. One of the earliest examples of a very competitive market in the United States was Minneapolis–St. Paul. During the 1980s, health plans began to concentrate their purchasing power through a series of mergers, up until the point that two large HMOs controlled 90 percent of the HMO market (Christianson et al. 1995). In response, hospital systems and multispecialty group practices began their own consolidation to retain bargaining power, until only three hospital networks controlled the bulk of hospital beds (National Health Policy Forum 1995).

More recently, San Diego has moved toward a great deal of consolidation. In order to retain bargaining power in a strong managed care environment (in which two-thirds of the population were in HMOs in

1995), the 44 hospitals in the city had consolidated so that five hospital systems accounted for over 90 percent of hospital admissions (*Los Angeles Times* 1995).

The ultimate effect of such consolidations is difficult to predict; it depends in large part not only on the relative bargaining power of different market participants, but also on the importance consumers put on issues such as health plan premiums and quality of care. Thus far it appears that increased HMO penetration results in lower premiums, although these savings decline when there are few competing provider groups (Zwanziger and Melnick 1996). As will be discussed in Section 4.3.1, the effect on quality of care is not yet clear.

4.2.3 Do Firms Maximize Profits?

In otherwise competitive economies, the health area is often an exception, in that many of the providers operate on a nonprofit basis. This is particularly true in the hospital sector, where in the vast majority of countries, for-profit status is the exception rather than the rule. Even in the United States, only about 14 percent of short-term-stay hospitals operate on a for-profit basis (American Hospital Association 1994).

We will not focus on this issue here, however, since it has already been dealt with extensively in the literature. Rather, we briefly raise a different reason to doubt the profit-maximization assumption: managers in the health sector, like their counterparts elsewhere in the economy, may seek to fulfill objectives other than maximizing their firms' overall profits. Because there is a vast literature on this subject (e.g., the study of total quality management), no attempt will be made to review the literature. Nevertheless, a few points about this assumption should be made.

In the 1960s, economist Harvey Leibenstein (1966) coined the term *X-efficiency*. The use of this term signified his belief that factors other than those that economists usually considered—in sum, the "X" factor— had potentially very substantial effects on efficiency in the economy. To motivate his argument, Leibenstein reviewed previous work on the social cost of traditional economic inefficiency, such as monopolies and trade barriers, and showed that they tended to have only minuscule effects on social welfare.[18] He then showed that, in contrast, the X-factor often tended to have a huge effect on efficiency.

What, then, is the X-factor? It is essentially the fact that motivational factors affect how firms translate their inputs into outputs. Leibenstein wrote, "The simple fact is that neither individuals nor firms work as

---

18. Such studies had calculated the "welfare loss" that results from higher prices and lower outputs associated with these deviations from perfect competition.

hard, nor do they search for information as effectively, as they could. The search arises because the relation between inputs and outputs in *not* a determinate one" (p. 407).

Standard economic theory assumes that firms maximize profits. Although most owners of firms (often the shareholders in publicly traded companies) certainly *want* to maximize profits, they do not run the companies by themselves. Rather, they hire managers and other employees to carry out the day-to-day business. In economic lingo, the owners of the firm are the principals, and the hired employees are the agents. Agents, however, may pursue some very different goals than profit maximization in carrying out their jobs. For instance, they may prefer not to work as hard as they could, they may be too cautious, or they may even plot against other employees to work their way up the hierarchy.[19,20]

One especially relevant application of this theory concerns independent practice association (IPA)-type HMOs. In IPAs, the owners of the HMO and its principal agents, the physicians with whom the IPA contracts, are physically separated and may have quite different goals. As a result, it is necessary for IPAs to come up with motivational factors to get physicians to act in the company's interest, but this is difficult to do and could reduce the quality of care provided. This issue will be further considered in Section 4.3.1, on capitation and incentive reimbursement.

4.2.4 Are There Increasing Returns to Scale?

Generally in economic markets, there are constant or decreasing returns to scale in production. That is, when a firm expands the use of all inputs by a certain proportion, the corresponding increase in output is the same (constant) or less than (decreasing) the increase in input usage.

One important implication of constant or decreasing returns to scale is that there is no advantage for society in having a monopoly. This can be understood by supposing the opposite for a moment: imagine there are increasing returns to scale. In such a case, the average cost of production would decline as we move from many firms that each supply a fraction of the total output, to one firm that supplies all of the output. A society

---

19. The extent to which managers and employees can deviate from profit maximization depends, to some degree, on how easy it is for other firms to enter the market. If entry costs are high, then an existing firm will be able to tolerate a larger degree of inefficiency without being subjected to competition from new entrants.

20. Even if employees do strive to maximize profits, another theory, the "Peter Principle," posits that such employees will eventually rise through the hierarchy until they reach their "level of incompetence," where they will remain. (See Peter and Hull [1969].) Although written in a humorous style, the book's theme would appear to contain more than a grain of truth.

might therefore be better off in encouraging the monopolization of such an industry, along with the subsequent regulation of that monopoly to ensure that it did not take advantage of its monopoly status to charge too much, produce too little, or both. In contrast, if there were not increasing returns to scale, there would seem to be little advantage to encouraging monopolies.

In the United States, a possible case can be made for the existence of increasing returns to scale in the hospital sector, particularly with regard to the provision of particular services. Stephen Finkler (1979) conducted the classic study of this type, examining economies of scale in the provision of open-heart surgery in California in the 1970s. Using a methodology called component enumeration, he essentially observed exactly what hospital resources were necessary for performing additional open-heart surgical procedures. He found that the average costs of such procedures did not bottom out until a hospital had provided about 500 per year, but that only 3 percent of California hospitals provided that many services. Finkler calculated that, in 1975 dollars, the United States could have saved $400 million by *regionalizing* open-heart surgery—that is, by providing such surgery in a select few regional facilities. He further calculated that the resulting incremental travel and other inconvenience costs would have absorbed only 6 percent to 9 percent of the savings. He also noted that "[h]eart surgery is only the tip of the iceberg" (p. 270).

Another aspect of increasing returns to scale in the hospital sector that is perhaps more often overlooked concerns health outcomes from surgery. One area of agreement among most health services researchers is that hospitals and physicians that have more experience in providing surgical services tend to obtain better health outcomes for their patients. One of the earliest studies of this type found that hospitals that performed over 200 operations per year of a particular type had mortality rates 25 percent to 41 percent lower than lower-volume hospitals, after controlling for case-mix differences (Luft, Bunker, and Enthoven 1979). A more recent study found that, when coronary artery bypass operations were done by high-volume surgeons in high-volume hospitals, mortality rates were 38 percent lower (Hannan et al. 1991). These results are also an indication of increasing returns to scale, in that quality is one of the chief outcomes in the hospital market.

Thus, in the health area, and especially for hospitals, there is much evidence to indicate the existence of increasing returns to scale. As will be discussed in Section 4.3.3, this has some important implications for the regulation of the hospital market.

4.2.5 Is Production Independent of the Distribution of Wealth?

A final assumption of the conventional economic model noted here is considered only rarely by economists, but is very important. That is the assumption that production is not related to the distribution of wealth.[21] Typically, firms are assumed to face *production functions* that look like Equation 4.2:

$$Q = f(L, K), \tag{4.2}$$

where Q is the quantity of output over some period of time, and L and K are the quantities of labor and capital inputs over that same period. The term f indicates the state-of-the-art technology that is used to transform these inputs into output. What the conventional model assumes is that this function f is unaffected by the way in which Q is distributed among the population.

Alternatively, what if this is not the case, and the distribution of output affects productivity? This would seem to be plausible. If people are poorly fed, then they are less likely to be productive workers. In a developed economy like the United States, where malnutrition is less widespread, the dependence of productivity on distribution would still hold in the following way. On average, poor people tend to be less educated and also tend to have more problematic health behaviors, which in turn reduces their health status. In a series of studies on the subject, Harold Luft (1973, 1978) found a causal relationship in which low socio-economic status resulted in lower health status, which in turn led to lower productivity, particularly among people with chronic conditions. Some health implications of this relationship are discussed in Section 4.3.4.

4.3 Implications for Health Policy

This chapter has attempted to show that the typical, passive role generally attributed to suppliers in competitive markets does not appear to apply very well to the field of health services. We questioned the validity of five assumptions of the competitive market, perhaps the most important of which, for our purposes, is that supply and demand are independently determined. In this section we discuss several ways in which relaxation of these assumptions results in a number of important implications concerning how suppliers' behavior can be influenced.

---

21. For a succinct discussion of this assumption, see Graaff (1971).

4.3.1 Capitation and Incentive Reimbursement

One of the key implications of the demand-inducement literature is that physicians can and do influence patients' decisions in a way that results in the provision of too many, and/or more complex, services. But physicians' ability to induce patient demand does not, by itself, mean that more services will be provided. A necessary corollary is that physicians are also paid more for providing more services—which is what happens when they are reimbursed on a fee-for-service basis. To see this, suppose that physicians had the ability to induce demand but were not paid more for each service they provided. In such a case, they would have no financial incentive to provide more services, even if they had the ability to do so.

It is this interaction between payment method and demand inducement that provides one of the key motivations for capitated payment systems. Under a fully capitated system, providers receive a fixed payment over a set period of time regardless of how many services they provide. Thus, they have no direct economic incentive to provide additional services. In fact, the incentive is the opposite; if they provide fewer services, profits will be higher since the capitation rate is unrelated to the number of services provided. Of course, if caregivers provide too few services, quality will be inhibited, providers may face possible lawsuits, and patients will likely become dissatisfied and move elsewhere.

The issues surrounding capitation and other forms of incentive reimbursement are fairly extensive, and they are complicated by the fact that these payment methods may apply to both health plans (e.g., insurers, HMOs) and providers. The following two subsections focus on these two groups separately.

Other supply-side measures that have been adopted to control costs are not reviewed here because they do not add any additional insights to the arguments being made. Some references are given to those wishing to pursue these topics: diagnosis-related groups (DRGs),[22] utilization review,[23] and practice guidelines.[24] A few broader supply-side measures used outside of the United States, such as technology controls and global budgeting, are presented later, in Section 4.3.3.

---

22. For a good review of the results of many DRG studies, see Coulam and Gaumer (1991).

23. For a review of the literature on second-opinion surgery, see Lindsey and Newhouse (1990). Useful studies on preadmission certification requirements for hospital stays include Wickizer, Wheeler, and Feldstein (1989), and Scheffler, Sullivan, and Ko (1991).

24. At the time of writing, little research had been published that evaluated the effect of practice guidelines on health costs. For background information on such guidelines, see Institute of Medicine (1990) and U.S. General Accounting Office (1991).

Paying Health Plans

In the United States, working-age individuals who have health insurance coverage usually obtain it through an employer. Typically, the employer contracts with several *health plans* to provide care to enrollees, although some employers choose a single plan for all employees. Health plans include so-called *indemnity*[25] *insurers* such as nonprofit Blue Cross and Blue Shield plans or for-profit commercial insurers, HMOs, and preferred provider organizations. In recent years, however, there has been much organizational innovation, so that the lines between these health plans have been blurred. For example, conventional insurers now often offer both indemnity insurance and HMO coverage, and HMOs often offer "point-of-service" benefits that allow members to go to out-of-network providers and still receive some reimbursement of the costs, as would be the case in fee-for-service coverage.

HMOs are almost always paid by employers on a capitation basis—a fixed amount of money per person per time period. One of the most important policy questions in the field of health economics is, "How much money do HMOs save over fee-for-service medicine?" One would expect some savings because, by being paid on a capitation basis, HMOs have a strong financial incentive to spend less. Although it is generally agreed that there are savings, a great deal of controversy is voiced about exactly how much. Estimates vary from as low as 4 percent to as much as 25 percent.[26] The true savings certainly lie somewhere in between, and probably depend on several factors, such as the type of HMO (group versus individual physician practice) and geographic area.

Because of the cost-savings potential of HMOs, many policymakers have been very favorably disposed toward them. Most recent proposals for U.S. health reform have relied on HMOs to achieve substantial savings. The concern, of course, is whether these cost savings come at the expense of unacceptable reductions in the quality of care provided.

One should not underestimate the tremendous power of the incentives that underlie capitation. To understand the stark differences between fee-for-service and capitation, it is useful to use an analogy.

---

25. Strictly speaking, these companies rarely sell true indemnity insurance. Under a true indemnity scheme, the insurer pays a fixed dollar amount per covered illness event (e.g., $50 for a visit to a doctor). Because such policies put the policyholder at much financial risk, insurers long ago found that *service benefits*, in which the policy pays a portion or all of the costs of a particular service, are more popular. Nevertheless, the term "indemnity insurance" is often used to distinguish conventional fee-for-service insurance from HMOs and preferred provider organizations.

26. The low-end estimates are from reviews of the literature conducted by the Congressional Budget Office (1994). The high-end numbers are from the RAND Health Insurance Experiment (Manning et al. 1984).

Being paid by fee-for-service is like getting a signed check from someone where the amount of the check has not been filled in; the incentive for the provider is to do more to get more. Capitation, however, is like getting a signed check where the amount has already been filled in. Since the provider already has the money, and is not going to get any more if it performs more services, the incentive is to do less in order to profit more.

The concern about quality under capitation is heightened when there is additional competition among HMOs. As HMOs compete against each other for employers to offer them and consumers to choose them, they need to cut their costs in order to keep their premiums competitive—and, by and large, they have done so (Zwanziger and Melnick 1996; Christianson et al. 1995). But if consumers do not have sufficient knowledge to determine which plans offer the best quality, as was argued in Sections 3.2.2 and 3.3.4, the cuts that HMOs make are more likely to reduce the quality of care provided.

Much research is being conducted on quality of care in HMOs versus fee-for-service medicine, the results of which are still far from certain. Most of the research up until now has concerned patient satisfaction, one component of quality but perhaps not as convincing as looking at health outcomes.[27] In general, it appears that HMOs do better than fee-for-service in terms of satisfaction with keeping costs down and in coordinating care among different physicians, but do worse with regard to continuity of care (e.g., seeing the same doctors), providing access to care (e.g., waiting times, or providing care at off-hours or on short notice), and perceptions about both the technical and personal side of care (Safran, Tarlov, and Rogers 1994; Rubin et al. 1993).

To most analysts, the more important issue is how HMOs have affected patients' medical outcomes. Although published research on this topic is still somewhat limited, it is growing quickly. A review of the literature through the early 1990s reported that most studies up until that time had found comparable quality between HMOs and fee-for-service medicine for various process and outcome measures of quality (Miller and Luft 1994), although some more recent evidence raises particular concern about how well the poor and elderly fare in HMOs (Ware et al. 1996).

Much more research on health outcomes in HMOs, other types of managed care systems, and fee-for-service is currently being conducted. It will be particularly interesting to see the results of future studies, as the periods under investigation will correspond to time periods in which there will have been much more competition in the HMO market. It is

---

27. This issue—whether a health system should be judged based on improving patients' health or on increasing their utility or satisfaction—is discussed at greater length in Chapter 5.

difficult to predict just how that may alter the quality findings. On the one hand, more competition could improve quality if that is the primary basis on which health plans compete, and if consumers are perceived as savvy judges of the quality of care provided. On the other hand, health plans, which are under extreme competitive pressures to control premiums, might cut resource use enough to result in reduced quality of care.

The material in this subsection might strike the reader as rather unsurprising. This is because nearly all health economists agree on the different incentives of capitation versus fee-for-service payment. What may generate more disagreement is exactly *why* these are important issues. What we posit here is that the reason we even consider capitation is that the marketplace for health services deviates so far from the competitive model that traditional, demand-side policy tools are largely inadequate. This issue is further pursued in Section 4.3.2, where we consider the issue of patient cost-sharing, the primary demand-side policy lever.

Paying Providers of Care

The previous subsection discussed how health plans tend to respond to payment incentives, but with a little reflection it should be clear that health plans cannot do it alone. A health plan does not provide care; rather, doctors and other providers do. A health plan that is paid on a capitation basis must find ways to get doctors to act to conserve resources, in order to keep plan premiums competitive.

Section 4.2.3 introduced the term "X-efficiency" to indicate that other factors besides those usually considered in microeconomics—most notably, ways in which a firm motivates its employees—are necessary for firms to be successful. In the HMO arena, this issue becomes especially important. The problem typically is not as great for group- and staff-model HMOs, which either employ their own physicians or contract with a medical staff as a whole. These HMOs tend to pay physicians a salary, which means that the physicians do not have a personal financial incentive to provide additional, marginally useful services. Nevertheless, such HMOs often also include incentive clauses to help ensure that the physicians consider the HMO's finances when making clinical decisions (Gold et al. 1994).

Compared to IPAs, group- and staff-model HMOs have a big advantage in this regard: physicians work in a common setting with a *corporate culture*. Such HMOs have any number of levers to help ensure that the medical staff act in a manner that is in the company's overall interest. Besides salary and capitation, such levers would include promotion within the organization, scheduling issues, and a variety of disciplinary actions, to name a few.

The problem faced by the HMO in influencing physicians' behavior is much greater in IPAs. Because physicians work in their own offices, and because they treat the patients from many HMOs as well as fee-for-service patients—not just a single IPA—it is difficult if not impossible to instill in these physicians any corporate culture. In addition, because they practice away from the HMO setting, the physicians have no direct oversight.

The IPA has an enormous problem. It obviously needs physicians in order to treat enrollees, but it has almost no control over these physicians. How can it motivate physicians to act in a way to conserve resources, so that the IPA can keep its cost below its capitation payments? Early IPAs were unsuccessful in this regard, and analysts expressed skepticism that such IPAs were able to control costs.[28] Such skepticism did not go away quickly; in 1994, the Congressional Budget Office (1994) reviewed existing literature and concluded that

> IPAs that have typical cost-sharing requirements [produce savings] that range from nothing to 9 percent, depending on how the IPAs are managed. Maximum savings would be credited for IPAs that select cost-conscious providers, maintain an effective network for inflation and control, place providers at financial risk, and generate a substantial portion of each provider's patient load. No savings would be credited for IPAs that accept all willing providers and that pay fee-for-service providers who do not share the risk. (p. 21)

It is very difficult to know just how much IPAs save compared to other HMOs or fee-for-service providers because conducting such comparative studies is difficult. With the exception of the RAND Health Insurance Experiment in the 1970s and early 1980s, in which people were randomly assigned to a single, staff-model HMO, researchers are plagued by the problem of *selection bias*.[29] This means that some health plans end up enrolling members who are either healthier or sicker than the rest of the population. Thus, the fact that IPAs might have lower costs than fee-for-service medicine may be a result of true cost savings, or alternatively, it may be due to the fact that they tend to have healthier enrollees. Although statistical techniques exist to help correct for this problem, the data available are rarely sufficient to fully solve it.

Some of the more recent literature is beginning to show that IPAs may be able to achieve the same sort of savings as group- and staff-model

---

28. For an analysis of HMOs before 1980, see Luft (1981).

29. There is a vast literature on the issue of selection bias. A good policy perspective appears in Newhouse (1994).

HMOs. For example, findings from the Medical Outcomes Study—which examined 20,000 patients in about 350 physician practices in 1986—found that prepaid multispecialty groups had hospitalization rates and ancillary test expenses that were less than those of traditional HMOs (Greenfield et al. 1992).

How, then, are IPAs overcoming some of their inherent disadvantages regarding cost control? The main way is likely to be through a strong physician motivational factor—incentive reimbursement. Early IPAs generally paid physicians on a fee-for-service basis, which gave them no incentive to control costs. But more recently, IPAs have adopted payment methods to help ensure that member physicians feel financial incentives similar to the HMO as a whole.

A variety of payment incentives exist.[30] Physicians can be paid by salary, capitation, and fee-for-service, and within these, there can be bonuses for meeting certain productivity or cost-containment goals. One common method is to withhold a certain amount of a primary physician's capitation fee, which is returned only if certain goals regarding low referral and hospitalization rates are met. Such incentives can also be tied to the ordering of diagnostic tests and radiological procedures.

Data from a survey of HMOs in 1994 indicate that, among IPAs, 56 percent use capitation as their principal payment method for primary care physicians, and 84 percent share financial risk with providers in some fashion. Most IPAs base these incentive payments on utilization and cost measures, as well as on quality indicators and consumer surveys. Specialists are also commonly paid on an incentive basis in IPAs, although this practice is not quite as common as for primary care physicians. Twenty percent of IPAs typically capitate their specialists, and 54 percent share financial risk with providers (Gold et al. 1994).

Although there has not been a great deal of research on the impact of these incentives, most studies find them to be at least somewhat effective, and sometimes very effective, in controlling HMO utilization and expenditures. In one study of Wisconsin employees enrolled in an IPA, a change from fee-for-service to capitation payment (with physicians sharing in the financial risk of hospitalization and specialty costs) resulted in an 18 percent increase in primary care visits, along with a 45 percent decline in referrals to specialists outside of the IPA. In addition, there was a 16 percent decrease in hospital admissions and a 12 percent drop in length of stay (Stearns, Wolfe, and Kindig 1992).

---

30. For a list and discussion of these methods, see: Hillman, Pauly, and Kerstein (1989); Hillman, Welch, and Pauly (1992); and Welch, Hillman, and Pauly (1990).

Similarly, in a study of an Illinois IPA, physicians were switched from fee-for-service payment with a 15 percent withhold (returned at end of year if utilization is kept below a target) to capitation payment with bonuses for reduced hospitalization and shared financial risk for specialty referral costs. It was found that specialist costs increased 2 percent in the year after the change, after rising by 12 percent in the previous year. Hospital outpatient service costs declined 7 percent, after increasing 12 percent in the previous year. But there was little change in inpatient hospital utilization (Ogden, Carlson, and Bernstein 1990).

On the international front, Mooney relates an interesting study on the power of incentive reimbursement. He reports on a study from Denmark in which physician payment methods were altered rather dramatically (Mooney 1994; Krasnik et al. 1990). In October 1987, general practitioners in Copenhagen changed from fully capitated payment to payment based partly on capitation and partly on fee-for-service, to conform with physicians in the rest of the country. This new system resulted in the ability of general practitioners (GPs) to make extra money for consultations, prescriptions, certain procedures and tests, and some other procedures. It was found that the provision of services that provided extra fees increased substantially together with and a large decrease in referrals to specialists and hospitals. From this, Mooney (1994) concludes that "[t]here clearly is considerable discretion on the part of GPs in how they act and remuneration systems can push them to go one way or another in how they treat their patients and whether they treat them themselves or refer them on in the system" (p. 127).

No studies currently exist that specifically examine how changing physician payment methods, per se, affects the quality of care provided (Rice and Gabel 1996). Without such studies, it is extremely difficult to address the overall question of whether patients and society are better off or not in a managed care environment. There is reason for concern, however: if physicians are given a financial incentive to cut back services, a plausible effect of that incentive is deteriorating quality.[31] In this regard, Marc Rodwin (1993) has written:

> Society makes a statement about the role of physicians when it provides incentives for them to help government or health care organizations reduce their costs. This is especially so if there are no equivalent financial incentives for physicians to improve quality of care. By using financial incentives to change the clinical practice of physicians, society calls forth self-interested

---

31. It must nevertheless be kept in mind that the fee-for-service system that is being replaced in the United States had its own problems—the main one being the provision of services that were unnecessary, or in some cases, harmful.

behavior. In asking physicians to consider their own interest in deciding how to act, we alter the attitude we want physicians ideally to have. For if physicians act intuitively to promote their patients' interests, we will worry less that they will behave inappropriately. But if their motivation is primarily self-interest, we will want their behavior to be monitored more carefully. (p. 153)

4.3.2 Issues Surrounding Patient Cost-Sharing

As noted several times in this book, the traditional economic method of trying to improve efficiency in the marketplace is to make patients pay more out-of-pocket for services. As may be recalled from Section 3.3.1, health insurance results in a societal "welfare loss" under the conventional model because people purchase services with a marginal benefit far below the cost of those services. Health economists therefore often are keen on increasing patient cost-sharing as a way of reducing this welfare loss (see Figure 3.6, above). This viewpoint was critiqued in Section 3.3.2.

In the United States, most employer-sponsored health insurance that is based on fee-for-service payments requires annual deductibles that averaged about $580 for a family in 1995, as well as a 20 percent coinsurance rate (Jensen et al. 1997; Gabel et al. 1994).[32] In addition, over 85 percent of HMOs also require cost-sharing in the form of copayments for each patient visit; in 1995, the typical amount was $10 (Jensen et al. 1997). Very few other countries employ substantial patient cost-sharing requirements for hospital and physician services, although many do for pharmaceuticals.[33]

In this section, we examine two issues associated with patient cost-sharing. The first part addresses problems in determining the effect of patient cost-sharing on controlling utilization and costs, while the second addresses equity. A further discussion of equity is included in Chapter 5.

The Effect of Patient Cost-Sharing on Utilization and Costs

The major study of patient cost-sharing, the RAND Health Insurance Experiment, concluded that patient cost-sharing was an effective method

---

32. There is nearly always an annual maximum amount for out-of-pocket costs, after which the insurer pays 100 percent of covered expenses. Recent surveys, however, do not report this information. In 1989, this typically ranged from $500 to $2,000 per year (Gabel et al. 1990).

33. One exception is France, where patients are required to pay 25 percent of physician fees and 20 percent of hospital per diem costs for stays up to 30 days in length. But many of the French are not subject to these copayment requirements—including the poor as well as disabled veterans and people suffering from any of 30 or so serious illnesses that can produce large hospital bills. Among those who are responsible for copayments, most purchase supplemental insurance coverage. Effectively, then, out-of-pocket costs are much lower in France than in the United States.

of reducing utilization and expenditures. People who had to pay 95 percent of charges had annual expenditures that were 28 percent less than those who paid nothing, and those with a 20 percent coinsurance rate had expenditures that were 18 percent less than those with free care (Manning et al. 1987). (See Table 3.1, in the previous chapter, for a summary of the results.) In addition, because the study also found little improvement in health outcomes among those with free care, study researchers concluded that comprehensive (i.e., first-dollar) national health insurance would be a wasteful way to spend a nation's resources (Newhouse et al. 1993).

Because the RAND study was the only major one that has used a true experimental design (i.e., random assignment of different types of insurance), it is the one that is normally used when making projections of the effect of patient copayments. Nevertheless, it should be recognized that the use of an experimental design jeopardizes the extent to which the results can be generalized to many health policy applications.

There are two major classifications of the *validity* of research studies: internal validity and external validity. Internal validity refers to how well study results accurately represent what actually occurred in the specific setting being examined. For example, suppose a researcher studied 50 IPAs and found that they resulted in a 15 percent reduction in expenditures. The extent to which this study is internally valid is measured by how accurate this result is compared to the true reduction in expenditures among that sample of IPAs. For a moment, let us say that this study was a good one, and that the findings appear to be reasonably accurate. But further suppose that the IPAs chosen were not representative of all IPAs because they were located on the West Coast. External validity refers to how well the results from a particular study can be generalized to other settings and/or populations.

It is generally agreed that the RAND Health Insurance Experiment was very strong in terms of its internal validity.[34] External validity is more of a concern, however. There are some commonly noted issues, such as the fact that the elderly were excluded and that the sample included only six sites in four states. Another such concern is whether the study, which was conducted from 1974 to 1982, is still timely. For example, during the 1980s alone, the number of hospital days fell by 38 percent per capita (U.S. Department of Health and Human Services 1992). If the study were conducted today, the results concerning the price responsiveness of hospital care might be much lower. Even if people had free care, they

---

34. Not everyone agrees with this, however. For some criticisms of the study, see Welch et al. (1987); and Hay and Olsen (1984). For responses to these criticisms by those who carried out the RAND study, see Newhouse et al. (1987); and Duan et al. (1984).

might not want, or might be prevented from obtaining, hospital care. There are also concerns about whether the findings with regard to health status would still hold, but such concerns are not directly relevant to the point being made here.

There is perhaps an even greater threat to the external validity of the RAND study's utilization and cost findings. To understand the issue, it is necessary to consider the experimental design in the RAND experiment. A random sample of individuals in six areas of the United States was chosen. Each site had an average of only about 1,000 study participants, many of whom were assigned to insurance plans that were equally generous as or more generous than those they had previously owned. Participants who were required to pay for care did indeed use fewer services. However, because only a small fraction of the population in each site participated— at most, 2 percent (Newhouse et al. 1993)—there would have been almost no effect on an individual physician's practice. Most doctors would have had, at most, only a handful of patients assigned to the high-coinsurance cells, so any reductions in service usage by those patients would not have markedly affected physician practice revenues. If everyone in an area had faced changing copayments—as might have occurred under various national health insurance proposals—the results could have been very different. Suppose that the plan called for coinsurance rates higher than the standard 20 percent level. Physicians might respond to the initial fall in business by inducing patient demand for services. This response could take the form of providing more follow-up services, more complex services, or even more surgery. The experiment examined only patient responses, not physician responses, to cost-sharing.

The converse may also be true. Suppose that a national health insurance plan removes all coinsurance. Subsequent demand may not rise as much as the RAND study would lead one to believe, for two reasons: (1) physicians may have less of a financial need than before to induce demand; and (2) governmental and private payors are likely to introduce other measures (e.g., tighter utilization review, expenditure targets, global budgeting) to quell the initial increase in patient demand.

The inability to deal with provider (and policymakers' regulatory) response in the RAND study has raised criticism since the inception of the experiment. In a discussion of these issues in 1974, when the experiment began, James Hester and Irving Leveson (1974) wrote,

> The utilization of health services is the result of a complex balancing between demand for health care and the supply system that provides it. While the changing needs of one individual or small group will not affect this overall balance, the large-scale shifts in quantity and source of medical care that

would result from a major national change in the financing of health care certainly would. Large changes in aggregate demand can be expected to produce substantial changes whose exact form is strongly influenced by specific administrative and financial regulations. . . . These changes will, in turn, feed back into the overall use patterns and costs, and influence again the users of the system. (pp. 53–54)

In response, Joseph Newhouse noted that the study was not "designed to replicate what would happen if various health insurance proposals were enacted into law," and furthermore, the study "deliberately selected sites that vary considerably with respect to the amount of stress on the delivery system" (Newhouse 1974, 236–37). That is, the six sites varied with respect to provider-to-population ratios.

A number of economists, although notably most of them from outside the United States, have provided similar criticisms of the generalizability of the RAND findings.[35] There has been little way of directly testing the issue, however.[36] Thus, it is safer to use the RAND study results as indicating the effect of cost-sharing on patients' demand for services (independent of any resulting provider response) rather than indicating ways in which overall utilization of services will change in response to large-scale policy initiatives concerning changes in patient cost-sharing.

Is Patient Cost-Sharing Equitable?

No matter how one defines equity—and several possible definitions will be discussed in Chapter 5—a strong case can be made that patient

---

35. See, for example, Evans (1984) and Mooney (1994). One U.S. economist who has made the same point is Alain Enthoven (1988), who wrote, "There are . . . problems in applying the results of the RAND experiment to national policy. RAND studied the behavior of about 7,700 people in six different cities. Thus, the proportion of the population affected by the experiment in any city was too small to have a noticeable effect on doctors' incomes, but the effects might be very different if everyone in a city were changed from a coverage with little co-insurance to one with a great deal. Initially, visits to the doctor would drop, but as the doctors found more time on their hands, all our experience suggests they would find other ways to make themselves useful: extra visits and consultations for hospitalized patients, more frequently advising patients who telephone that they should come in to be seen, and the like. What applies to a small sample might not apply to the whole community" (p. 17).

36. The only U.S. study that addresses this issue was from a small natural experiment that was analyzed by Marianne Fahs (1992), on the experience of one multispecialty group practice located in Appalachia in 1977. Fahs compared utilization in the year before the institution of cost-sharing with that during the two years following its institution, for two groups: mine workers who faced increasing cost-sharing requirements, and steel workers who did not. The study found that physicians responded to the imposition of cost-sharing on their mine worker patients by changing their practice behavior for their steel worker patients. Fahs concludes that "when the economic effects of cost-sharing on physician service use are analyzed for all patients within a physician practice, the findings are remarkably different from those of an analysis limited to those patients directly affected by cost-sharing" (pp. 25–26).

cost-sharing is inequitable. This is because of two interrelated issues: cost-sharing payments account for a greater proportion of income for those with lower income; and those with lower income tend to be sicker and to require more services. It should be obvious that families with lower incomes who do seek medical care will spend a greater proportion of their income in order to meet these cost-sharing requirements. Differences in wage and salary rates abound throughout the economy. The average wage of people with managerial and professional jobs, for example, is more than double that for those with service-related jobs. Even across industries, there are large differences; communication workers, for instance, make 50 percent more than construction workers. Black families are two-and-a-half times as likely as white families to have incomes less than $10,000 (U.S. Department of Commerce 1996).

This problem is accentuated when health status is taken into consideration. To give one example, in 1994, 20 percent of Americans with incomes less than $14,000 rated their health as "fair" or "poor," compared to only 4 percent with incomes above $50,000 (U.S. Department of Health and Human Services 1997).

The issue of the distributional burden of cost-sharing is well summarized by Robert Evans and his colleagues, who have written about what would occur if the tax-financed Canadian health system were to institute patient cost-sharing:

> The primary effect of substituting user fees for tax finance is *cost shifting*—the transfer of the burden of paying for health care from taxpayers to users of care. . . . [P]eople pay taxes in rough proportion to their incomes, and use health care in rough proportion to their health status or need for care. The relationships are not exact, but in general sicker people use more health care, and richer people pay more taxes. It follows that when health care is paid for from taxes, people with higher incomes pay a larger share of the total cost; when it is paid for by the users, sick people pay a larger share. . . . Whether one is a gainer or loser, then, depends upon where one is located in the distribution of both income . . . and health. . . . In general, a shift to more user fee financing redistributes net income . . . from lower to higher income people, and from sicker to healthier people. The wealthy and healthy gain, the poor and sick lose. (Evans, Barer, and Stoddart 1993, 4)

Although the RAND Health Insurance Experiment did not find too many instances in which reduced patient cost-sharing improved health status, there was evidence of such an effect for those with lower income. Some examples:

- Low-income families at elevated risk benefited the most from free care. The reduction in diastolic blood pressure among lower-income persons who were judged to be at an elevated risk for hypertension was 3.3 mm Hg, compared to only 0.4 mm Hg for similar people with higher incomes (Brook et al. 1983).

- Low-income persons in poor health who were given free care had the largest reduction in serious symptoms (Shapiro, Ware, and Sherbourne 1986).

- Among children of poor families who were at the highest risk, those with free care were less likely to have anemia than those in the cost-sharing plans (Valdez 1986).

Additional evidence also comes from looking at how coinsurance affected the receipt of general medical examinations. Low-income adults in the cost-sharing groups received 46 percent fewer exams than their counterparts with free care, compared to only a 29 percent reduction for other groups. For the children of those with cost-sharing, the figures were 32 percent and 21 percent fewer exams, respectively (Lohr et al. 1986). Finally, the RAND study examined the influence of coinsurance on the probability of obtaining medical care that was judged to be highly effective at treating a particular episode of illness. Among nonpoor children, those who had to pay coinsurance were 85 percent as likely to obtain care as the nonpoor with free care. For poor children, however, cost-sharing was a much bigger deterrent to obtaining medical care judged to be highly effective for a particular illness episode. Compared to those with free care, poor children whose families faced coinsurance were only 56 percent as likely to receive services. A similar pattern, although not as marked, was found for adults (Lohr et al. 1986).

To only a limited extent does U.S. health policy deal explicitly with the equity problems arising from the burden of patient cost-sharing. The primary way is through the Medicaid program, which does not require patient copayments. However, Medicaid only actually covers 46 percent of the poor (U.S. Department of Commerce 1996).

Summary

Some of the problems with relying on patient cost-sharing have been summarized by Canadian economists Greg Stoddart and colleagues, who found four overriding reasons to eschew the implementation of cost-sharing in their own national health system:

1. charges do not lead to selective reductions in utilization of only unnecessary or less necessary services, but affect the utilization of needed services as well (while much ineffective care continues to be delivered);

2. the distribution effects—both financial and health effects—of charges are potentially quite serious for certain groups in the population,

especially as health care use becomes more concentrated within small and very ill segments of the population;

3. analyses of the effects of user charges must take into account the significant, offsetting response of suppliers to reductions in patient-initiated utilization; and

4. charges are neither a necessary nor a sufficient condition for overall cost control in health care systems. (Stoddart, Barer, and Evans 1993, p. 57)

There are some ways to try to ameliorate the equity problems. The present author, for example, was involved in formulating a proposal for U.S. health reform in which cost-sharing requirements were explicitly tied to patient income (Rice and Thorpe 1993). Such proposals would probably be difficult to enact, however, for both political and administrative reasons.[37] Other countries, therefore, have focused their efforts on alternative means of controlling expenditures, as described next.

4.3.3 Regulating Growth in the Health Sector

As noted earlier, few developed countries besides the United States rely on patient cost-sharing to control expenditures. This is not to say that they are indifferent to how much they are spending, however. Quite to the contrary: because government tends to be quite heavily involved in the financing of services, the health sector must compete against all others for funding. This tends to result in strong pressure to keep health expenditures in check.[38] This section will briefly outline some of the cost-containment strategies that other countries use. Readers interested in more specifics will need to study the delivery and financing systems of particular countries.

One can only go so far in generalizing how different countries have approached cost containment in the area of health. Because each country has a different system and faces different political barriers, no two countries are alike. There are, however, some common threads.

One of the most common methods of cost containment, especially for hospital and physician services, is the use of some kind of *global*

---

37. Perhaps the largest impediment is that the proposal relies on the income tax system to determine patient liabilities. This likely would result in people viewing cost-sharing as a tax, and taxes tend to be very unpopular.

38. Among developed countries, there is not a positive relationship between government involvement in health financing and the proportion of national income devoted to health (Jonsson 1989). Thus, at least on the surface, there does not appear to be a causal relation between more government and more spending. Nevertheless, one should use such figures with caution because so many other factors are correlated with both national income and government's involvement in financing of health services.

budgets. Global budgets "tend to be prospectively set caps on spending for some portion of the health care industry" (Wolfe and Moran 1993, 55). The exact meaning, however, varies from country to country. In some countries, such as Canada, hospitals receive an annual global budget to cover their entire operating budget.[39] In Germany, there are regional budgets for different types of physician services. A survey of nine European countries found that all used some form of global budgeting. Most studies of global budgeting have found that global budgets do help control spending (Wolfe and Moran 1993; U.S. General Accounting Office 1991; Abel-Smith 1992).

Cost control in other developed countries does not typically rest, however, with the national government. Rather, most countries rely on more regional constraints. As Bengt Jonsson (1989) has noted,

> The single most important lesson for the European health care systems during the 1980s concerns the role of central government. The European systems have been able to reduce the total costs of health care not so much through central planning and regulation as through global budgets at the regional level. . . . The reason for this is the obvious difficulty in managing such a huge and complicated system from the center. (p. 92)

Regional global budgeting has not been used in isolation, though. Most countries employ several different methods of containing costs. One of the most common is the control of the diffusion of medical technologies. As was shown earlier in Table 2.3, there tend to be far more of many medical technologies in the United States than in other countries. This is largely because the decisions to acquire such technologies are usually made by regional or national government in other countries, whereas each hospital or medical practice makes its own acquisition decisions in the United States (Jonsson 1989).

This has led to a much greater level of regionalization of hospital and surgical care. As discussed in Section 4.2.4, evidence from the United States indicates that quality can be higher, and costs lower, if services are concentrated in regional specialty centers to take advantage of various economies of scale. In Canada and Europe, this tends to be the case, with regional bodies responsible both for allocating the funds for new capital equipment and for holding the ultimate authority to approve such acquisitions.

Although it is harder to generalize about this area, one can also make a case that other countries save by stressing preventive care more so than is done in the United States. In part because it is easier to focus on

---

39. Capital expenses are paid for (and rationed) separately.

specific preventive services under a nationalized system, there appears to be more of an emphasis on such services in Europe than in the United States. One study of preventive care for children and pregnant women in six developed countries (Canada, Sweden, France, Germany, Japan, and the United Kingdom) found that

> [d]espite wide variations in financing mechanisms, levels of health care spending, and cost containment strategies among these six systems, each provides comprehensive services to all children and pregnant women. Additionally, access and outcome measures . . . are better than those of the United States. (Chaulk 1994, 7)

This was due, in large measure, to comprehensive and accessible prenatal and infant and child care.

In addition, administrative costs are higher in the United States than in other countries. Substantial savings can be garnered by guaranteeing coverage to all citizens and by removing most of the paperwork involved in the billing process. For example, the cost of administering the Canadian health system represents only about 0.1 percent of the country's gross national product, far less than the 0.6 percent figure for the United States (Evans 1990).

But these may not be the primary reasons that other countries (all with national health insurance systems) appear to generate savings. Rather, as Evans has argued in a number of papers comparing the Canadian and U.S. experiences, it is due to government's *monopsony*[40] power over provider payments and over other aspects of the system such as technology diffusion (Evans 1990; Evans 1983). If the government provides the vast majority of payments, it has greater ability to control total health-related costs. Providers are unable to obtain additional revenues outside of the system if the system encompasses the entire population. This is the main reason why some analysts believe that providing health insurance coverage to the entire population actually results in savings.

This conclusion holds not only in Canada but in Europe as well, where Brian Abel-Smith (1992) concluded his analysis of European systems by stating,

> The main message from the experience of the European Community is that it is technically possible to control health care costs by government regulation of supply rather than demand, particularly by applying budgets to hospitals. . . . The key to Europe's success is the use of monopsony power whereby one purchaser dominates the market, and not just the hospital market. Where there are many purchasers, as in Germany, they are forced

---

40. A monopsony occurs when there is only one buyer of a particular product (here, medical care).

to act together. Because the insurers are not allowed more revenue, either from tax or contributions, and because what they can charge the insured in copayments is centrally determined, they are forced either to confront providers or to ration their allowable resources. In most countries this does not lead to lines of patients waiting for treatment. (p. 414)

Whether a government-financed national health insurance would help control costs in the United States is an open question, however. In fact, recent experience in the United States has shown that the movement toward managed care has succeeded in controlling U.S. costs. But even if there is a resurgence in these costs in the future, the issue arises about whether policies used successfully in other countries would work in the United States. One problem lies in generalizing from other countries' experiences. Returning to global budgets, if they were implemented in the United States, they might operate differently than they do elsewhere. One important point Abel-Smith (1992) makes is that, in other countries, there is less of an issue of regulators being influenced by the industry that they regulate.

The larger problem, however, is whether Americans *want* to change their health system. Although they show great dissatisfaction in surveys (Blendon et al. 1990), Americans might be even less happy with a different system. About half of Americans claim that the country currently spends *too little* on health services (Blendon et al. 1995b). Quite naturally, people may wish to avail themselves of many of the things—particularly, the possibility of a longer and better life—that could arise from additional spending.

In addition, constraints on spending can lead to types of rationing that may be viewed as undesirable, such as longer waits to obtain appointments or even surgical procedures.[41] In fact, when asked about national health insurance, Americans' support plummets (from 73 percent to 36 percent) if such insurance would result in longer waits to receive care (Blendon and Donelan 1990).[42]

It is therefore difficult to reach definitive conclusions about the applicability to the United States of other countries' experiences with regulating the supply side of the market for health services. Policy measures used by other countries do seem to have been successful historically.

---

41. There seems to be little agreement on the amount of so-called queuing for services in other countries. Data published on queuing in Ontario by the U.S. General Accounting Office (1991) showed the potential for significant waits for elective services, but did not pinpoint the magnitude of the problem because it published only minimum and maximum queues, not averages.

42. Interestingly, although Americans are less tolerant than Canadians about waiting for services, they seem to be more tolerant than Germans. For example, 28 percent of Canadians would be unwilling to wait more than one day for treatment of a suspected cracked rib, versus 42 percent of Americans and 59 percent of Germans (Blendon et al. 1995b).

But the failure of comprehensive reform of the health sector makes it difficult to envision enacting similar policies any time soon in the United States. It may be that an emphasis on market forces will continue to dominate U.S. health policy for some time to come, until (and if) sufficient dissatisfaction results from such a policy.

4.3.4 Improving Productivity by Providing Insurance

Despite their belief that additional health insurance results in a welfare loss to society, many if not most health economists believe that everyone should be provided at least some health insurance coverage. The basis of such a belief typically is from the viewpoint of equity or fairness; that is, for ethical reasons people should receive at least some level of coverage. It is less common to see health economists argue for universal, comprehensive health insurance coverage from an *efficiency* standpoint. (Such an argument was first introduced here in Section 3.3.1.)

One can also make a strong argument for providing health insurance coverage from an efficiency as well as an equity standpoint—especially for the poor. As alluded to in Section 4.2.5, a competitive market may underprovide health insurance coverage if poor income distribution results in the inability of some people to be as productive in the workplace as they might otherwise.[43]

This argument rests on three assumptions: (1) health insurance increases utilization; (2) greater utilization increases health status; and (3) better health status improves worker productivity. There is general agreement about the validity of propositions (1) and (3), but some doubt about (2).

Much of this doubt about proposition (2) comes from the RAND Health Insurance Experiment, where it was found that, among the nonelderly, care provided free of coinsurance and deductibles did little to improve health status among the nonelderly population (Brook et al. 1983; Keeler 1987).[44] But as discussed earlier in Section 4.3.2, other findings from the study indicated that poorer people did indeed benefit from free care.

The fact that programs such as Medicaid exist in the United States indicates a belief that poor people should be provided with health insurance so that they may be able to achieve up to their capabilities. The point here is that such an attitude can stem from efficiency as well as egalitarian considerations.

---

43. It is possible that an even greater improvement in health would occur if income distribution itself were more nearly equal, but as argued in Chapter 5, there is much stronger support for in-kind rather than in-cash transfer payments to the poor.

44. The study did not examine the elderly mainly because they already had Medicare coverage.

5

EQUITY AND REDISTRIBUTION

IT IS perhaps unfortunate to leave issues about equity and redistribution to the end of the book because this masks their importance. Although economists often focus on what is efficient, most people would appear to be more concerned about what is fair. In this regard, Daniel Hausman and Michael McPherson (1993) write, "Notions of fairness, opportunity, freedom, and rights are arguably of more importance in policy making than are concerns about moving individuals up their given preference rankings" (p. 676). Despite the importance of these issues, they have not received sufficient attention from health economists.

Section 5.1 provides a brief summary of ways in which traditional economic theory deals with the subject of the redistribution of wealth. Section 5.2 provides a critique of this theory, focusing on problems with "ordinal utilitarianism," the philosophy on which most policy conclusions are based. Section 5.3 then provides several applications of this critique to health policy.

5.1 The Traditional Economic Model

Although many economists have given considerable thought to the issues of equity and the redistribution of wealth, such issues play little part in the traditional microeconomic model. Rather than concerning itself with how people come into possession with their initial stock of wealth, the traditional model devotes nearly all of its attention to how they allocate the resources over which they have already been assigned property rights (Young 1994).

Figure 5.1   Edgeworth Box, Modified

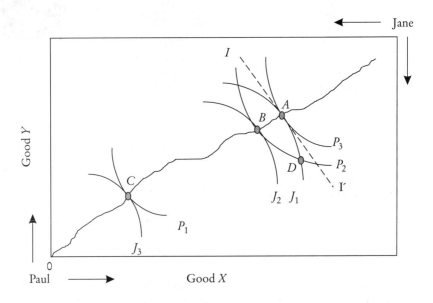

To recapitulate, we will reproduce the Edgeworth Box shown in Figure 2.7 with a few modifications to make Figure 5.1. For simplicity, we assume that there are only two goods produced by society (this time, called X and Y) and that there are only two consumers, Paul and Jane. We saw that any allocation of the two goods that falls along the contract curve $O–A$ is defined to be economically efficient because there are no reallocations that will make one of the consumers better off without making the other worse off. (Unlike in Chapter 2, we will ignore the issue of envy here.)

With the Edgeworth Box, we can see how any initial allocation of resources will be transformed, through trading, to a final equilibrium. To illustrate, suppose that Paul is initially endowed with about three-quarters of good X and just less than half of good Y (with Jane getting the remainder of each), which is depicted at point D. This is not a Pareto-optimal point because it is possible to make one or both of the consumers better off. Paul and Jane will therefore engage in trading, and afterward, the final allocation will fall along the contract curve somewhere between points A and B. The exact point depends on the relative bargaining skills of the two people.

Only one point on the contract curve will, however, also maximize *social* welfare. (See Section 2.1.4 for a discussion of social welfare functions.) To reach that point, the economic model assumes that society will engage in redistribution of the initial endowments of wealth so that this particular point on the contract curve will be reached after the market has reached an equilibrium through trading.

Thus, under the traditional model, competition is used to ensure that resources are being used efficiently. Wealth is redistributed, through money transfer payments (since in the real world there are numerous goods, not just two), to ensure that the final competitive equilibrium results in a distribution of resources that is in accordance with society's desires. (The issue of how to carry out such a redistribution through taxation, without marring the efficiency brought about by competition, is a major problem, but one that was already addressed in Sections 2.2.2 and 2.3.2.)

5.2 Problems with the Traditional Model

A number of criticisms have been leveled against the traditional model in terms of how it deals (or, perhaps more appropriately, does not deal) with equity and fairness, as well as with the distribution of resources. These objections share one common element: they dispute the notion of ordinal utilitarianism, on which the traditional model is based.

This section critiques two of the assumptions listed in Table 1.1:

Assumption 9.   Social welfare is based solely on individual utilities, which in turn are based solely on the goods and services consumed.

Assumption 15. The distribution of wealth is approved of by society.

5.2.1 Overview of Utilitarianism

Utilitarianism is the philosophy that assumes that social welfare is simply the sum or aggregate of all individuals' welfare. Under this philosophy, utility is a personal psychological perception, and, to the economist, it is based on the goods a person possesses.

As discussed in Section 3.1.1, early advocates of so-called classical utilitarianism such as Jeremy Bentham believed that these utilities not only could be quantified, but could also be added across individuals. Modern economics rebelled against such a concept, relying instead on the notion of *ordinal* rather than *cardinal utility*. Under ordinal utility, individuals choose which bundle of goods they prefer to any other instead of quantifying how much utility is derived from one bundle versus another.[1]

---

1. Some critics, however, believe that modern economists have gone too far in eschewing interpersonal comparisons of utility. Little (1957), for example, claims that most people are able

One needs to be careful in discussing utilitarianism because the term encompasses a number of seemingly distinct beliefs.[2] As noted, under classical utilitarianism, individual utilities can be quantified using a metric that is consistent across individuals. Ordinal utilitarianism, on which modern theory is based, requires only that individuals be able to rank alternative bundles of goods (which allows economists to employ indifference curves). But there are other utilitarian concepts as well. Under incremental utilitarianism, goods should be put in the hands of those who accrue the most gain from them. And one hybrid form of utilitarianism allows intensity of preference to come into play (e.g., one good brings three times as much utility as another to a person), but does not permit utilities to be added across individuals.[3]

We have noted that economic theory is based on the concept of ordinal utilitarianism. In support of this concept, Kenneth Arrow (1983), a strong advocate of the use of ordinal utility in evaluating social welfare, has stated that

> [t]he implicit ethical basis of economic policy judgment is some version of utilitarianism. At the same time, descriptive economics has relied heavily on a utilitarian psychology in explaining the choices made by consumers and other economic agents. The basic theorem of welfare economics—that under certain conditions the competitive economic system yields an outcome that is optimal or efficient . . . —depends on the identification of the utility structures that motivate the choices made by economic agents with the utility structures used in judging the optimality of the outcome of the competitive system. As a result, the utility concepts which, in one form or another, underlie welfare judgments in economics as well as elsewhere . . . have been subjected to an intensive scrutiny by economists. (p. 97)

What Arrow is saying is that the belief that competition results in socially desirable outcomes hinges on:

- individuals making choices that maximize their well-being; and
- society evaluating its own well-being solely on the basis of the utility enjoyed by its individuals.

Chapter 3 was devoted, in large part, to examining the first bulleted point. Much of the present critique will focus on the second.

---

to make valid judgments about whether one person is happier than another, or gets a greater amount of utility than another person from a particular good.

2. For a discussion of the different types of utilitarianism, see Elster (1992).

3. Elster (1992) has coined this as "Neumann-Morgenstern utility," after the founders of game theory.

5.2.2 Problems with Ordinal Utilitarianism

This section explores three problems with the concept of utilitarianism employed by modern economics, each of which has important implications concerning equity and the distribution of wealth. The first problem concerns lack of breadth; the concept ignores issues of social justice and fairness. The second problem concerns lack of depth; utilitarianism is defined solely in terms of a single, goods-based, psychological metric, ignoring other potentially important conceptions of what drives individual and social welfare. The third problem is perhaps more practical; utilitarianism mistakenly assumes that the socially optimal redistribution of wealth should take the form of cash grants rather than transfers of the goods and services themselves.

Social Justice and Fairness

Modern economics in general, and utilitarianism in particular, do not concern themselves with what is right or fair. Rather, the possession of goods brings utility to individuals and therefore to society, which is conceived of as simply the aggregate of all individuals.

No concern is given to whether or not the overall distribution of wealth is *justified*. This is not to say that issues of income distribution are ignored. In fact, the people in a society may indeed be concerned about distributional issues and may choose to tax the rich to provide for the poor. But if that occurs, it is the result of social choice (as exemplified by the social welfare function) and not necessarily based on social justice.

To understand this distinction—a crucial one—it is useful to consider the difference between altruism and equity. The former is based on preferences, for example, I want the poor to have more so I provide donations or vote to increase taxes. Thus, providing for the poor makes *me* better off because their welfare enters my utility function. In contrast, according to Adam Wagstaff and Eddy van Doorslaer (1993),

> Social justice (or equity), on the other hand, is not a matter of preference. As [Anthony] Culyer puts it: " . . . the source of value for making judgements about equity lies outside, or is extrinsic to, preferences. . . . The whole point of making a judgement about justice is so to frame it . . . independently of interests of the individual making it." Social justice thus derives from a set of principles concerning what a person ought to have *as a right*. (p. 8)

The issue of what people should have as a right is obviously a controversial one, and one that has held the attention of philosophers and economists alike. As noted, traditional economic theory, as based on an ordinal view of utilitarianism, sidesteps this issue; rights do not come into play except insofar as society has defined property rights. But how such property rights are assigned is not part of the purview of economics; rather, it is a societal decision based, presumably, on other considerations.

As might be imagined, different philosophers (and economists) have reached different conclusions about what things people should have as a right. At one extreme, Robert Nozick (1994) has proposed a libertarian philosophy in which the distribution of wealth is just if: (1) the original assignment of wealth was arrived at fairly, and (2) the current distribution was arrived at through voluntary exchange. However, whether the original distribution was arrived at in a "just" fashion is certainly a matter of opinion; as a result, this philosophy has been aptly coined as one of "finders keepers" (Elster 1992; Stone 1996).

The best-known modern exposition of social justice and rights is the book by John Rawls (1971), *A Theory of Justice*. The next two subsections will describe and critique Rawls's viewpoint.

Rawls's Theory

Rawls's theory, which he calls "justice as fairness," provides an alternative to utilitarian philosophy. To determine what is fair, he invokes a concept called the "original position," in which people choose the principles of a just society from a position where "no one knows his place in society, his class position or social status, nor does any one know his fortune in the distribution of natural assets and abilities, his intelligence, strength, and the like" (Rawls 1971, 12).

In addition, one does not know the sort of society in which he or she will be placed; it may be a democracy or, alternatively, a dictatorship in which there is a small ruling class, with the rest of the population assigned to slavery. Rawls calls this lack of information about one's talents and standing, a "veil of ignorance." His goal is to determine the system of justice that rational, self-oriented people would choose when placed in the original position.

The other term that needs definition is "primary goods," which are defined as "rights and liberties, powers and opportunities, income and wealth" (p. 62). Self-respect turns out to be another key primary good.

Rawls posits that people in the original position would accept the proposition that primary goods should "be distributed equally unless an unequal distribution of any, or all, of these values is to everyone's advantage. Injustice, then, is simply inequalities that are not to the benefit of everyone" (p. 62).

The punch line—the system of justice that Rawls believes would be adopted by a society whose members consider these issues under the veil of ignorance in the original position—is what he calls the "difference principle." Under the difference principle, society is better off only when it makes its least well-off people better off. In other words, society's

Figure 5.2   Social Welfare under Rawls's Theory

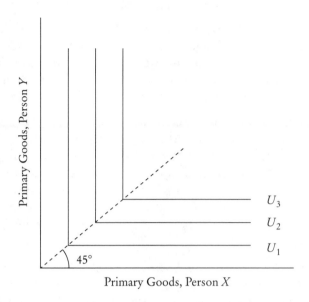

Source: Reprinted by permission of the publisher from *A Theory of Justice* by John Rawls, Cambridge, Mass.: Havard University Press, Copyright © 1971 by the President and Fellows of Harvard College.

resources should be devoted to increasing the primary goods possessed by the most disadvantaged people. The only time that resources will go to the group that does not occupy the bottom rung is when by doing so, benefits will trickle down to the most disadvantaged group.

This result—that in the original position, people will adopt the above method of allocating primary goods—is called "maximin."[4] In essence, people will choose to maximize the lot of those who have the minimum. The unusual nature (at least to an economist) of this philosophy can be seen from Figure 5.2, which shows a set of social indifference curves under the theory. Let the x-axis be the primary goods enjoyed by person X, and the y-axis those enjoyed by person Y. Each curve shows distributions that are, from society's viewpoint, equally desirable. Higher curves (i.e., those farther from the origin) represent higher levels of social welfare. The 45° line shows equal distributions of primary goods.

The indifference curves are L-shaped; society is no better off when Y has more primary goods if those possessed by X do not increase. The only way to increase social welfare—that is, to get on a higher indifference curve—is to provide more to the person who has the least.

---

4. This stands for *maximum minimorum*.

Why would people, placed in the original position, come up with such a conception of justice? Rawls has a simple answer:

> Since it is not reasonable for [a person] to expect more than an equal share in the division of social goods, and since it is not rational for him to agree to less, the sensible thing for him to do is to acknowledge as the first principle of justice one requiring an equal distribution. Indeed, this principle is so obvious that we would expect it to occur to anyone immediately. (pp. 150–51)

Before moving on to a critique of Rawls's theory, it is necessary to note its policy implications. Although the theory is abstract and cannot be applied directly to many problems,[5] there is one overriding implication: society should engage in far more redistribution than it currently does. This is because many, if not most, redistributive programs are not targeted solely at those who are worst off in society. In fact, one could argue that relatively little goes to this group. In this regard, Gordon Tullock (1979) has written,

> So far as I know there is absolutely no reason to believe that majority voting or any of the variants of democratic government transfer an "optimal" amount. Indeed, I would argue that they do very badly, since the bulk of the transfers they generate are transferred back and forth within the middle class; and, so far as I know, there are no arguments that would indicate that these transfers are desirable. (p. 172)

Although Rawls did not list health as one of the primary goods, some analysts have disagreed with this decision. According to Ronald Green (1976), "Access to health care is not only a social primary good, but possibly one of the most important such goods [because] disease and ill health interfere with our happiness and undermine our self-confidence and self-respect" (p. 120). The types of services that would be included as part of a universal health plan would include such things as "basic preventive and therapeutic services" (Green 1986, 120).[6]

Critique of Rawls's Theory

Although Rawls's theory is usually praised even by its critics, a number of objections have been leveled against it. Here we discuss three of them.

People Would Not Choose Maximin.

Rawls assumes that rational people would choose the maximin principle to distribute primary goods. Many analysts, particularly economists, disagree, claiming that to reach this conclusion, one must assume a huge amount of risk aversion among

---

5. See Elster (1992) for a more thorough discussion of this criticism.
6. For more views on this topic, see Daniels (1985).

the population. To illustrate, suppose that people were asked to choose between two alternative societies, one in which 95 percent of the people were endowed with $10,000 in resources and the other 5 percent with $1,000; and another in which everyone was endowed with $1,500. It seems unlikely that most people would choose the latter—but that is what Rawls predicts. Indeed, survey research on how people claim they would behave under the original position indicates that they would prefer the first scenario, so long as they did not view the $1,000 as too low for subsistence. In general, when asked, people seem to choose to maximize average income subject to some minimum constraint or floor, rather than the maximin solution (Miller 1992).

In fairness to Rawls, however, there are two responses to the above argument. First, Rawls makes it clear that under the original position, one does not know the kind of society in which one would be placed. It is entirely possible that it would be dictatorial, with almost all wealth lavished on a few and the rest of the populace living in poverty. Given that uncertainty, it is easier to see how one would come up with maximin—if there is a risk of being a member of the (subjugated) masses, why not choose a system of justice in which resources are equally distributed? In surveys that have been conducted, it is very likely that people would have imagined themselves placed within a democratic society like the one they were used to.

Second, although one could argue that Rawls's theory will result in unreasonable choices "on paper," it may be that such odd results are unlikely to come about under real-world circumstances. In the above example, the implication is that, somehow, the subjugation of 5 percent of the population will allow the other 95 percent to accrue far more wealth. In this regard, Rawls (1971) states, "[I]t seems extraordinary that the justice of increasing the expectations of the better placed by a billion dollars, say, should turn on whether the prospects of the least favored increase or decrease by a penny" (p. 157). This is indeed unlikely; testing the validity of the theory using these kinds of numbers might in itself be unfair. Nevertheless, there is an issue about whether Rawls's theory might sacrifice too much efficiency to gain a small amount of equity.

More Groups Should Receive Favorable Treatment. Under Rawls's theory, the only group that receives a greater portion of primary goods is the one that is worst off. This is not necessarily desirable—why not help the nearly worst off at the same time you are helping the worst off; might not that be what people would choose in the original position? (Sen 1982). In addition, some people might not fully enjoy or use the primary goods that they are transferred and that others might need more than others in order to enjoy life. These issues, which are explored in the next section, are not dealt with through the application of Rawls's theory (Sen 1982).

This raises a related issue: How do we know who is worst off? In the theory, Rawls uses a "representative person" within each subgroup of society. The problem is that some of these representative people may be better off in some characteristics and worse off in others. If that is the case, who would be assigned the first primary goods to be redistributed? Furthermore, if one looks at the way in which decisions are made in society, then it is clear that all aspects of a person's background are not considered in distributing scarce resources. To give one example in the literature, the fact that you do not get a scarce kidney for transplantation (and therefore must remain on dialysis) will not typically increase your chances of being admitted to a university over other qualified candidates (Young 1994). Societal decision making is typically done on a "local" rather than "global" basis (Elster 1992; Young 1994). In the above example, those who decide on college admissions do not also decide on kidney allocation, nor do they usually consider such factors.

Other Factors Should Form the Basis of Reallocation.   This material will be mentioned only briefly to avoid repeating what is in the next section, which examines other conceptions of welfare (besides those in utilitarianism). Just as utilitarianism is limited in its conception of ways in which resources should be distributed, so, it can be argued, is Rawls's theory.

In the theory, the only basis for redistribution is where a person stands in society with respect to his or her possession of primary goods. This viewpoint would appear to be rather limited for a number of reasons, two of which are listed here:

- Under the theory, people are entitled to an equal share of resources irrespective of their work effort, motivation, and so on. This is because what a person is born with is, according to Rawls, really just the result of a "natural lottery," which "is arbitrary from a moral perspective." As a result, he believes that "[e]ven the willingness to make an effort, to try, and so to be deserving in the ordinary sense is itself dependent on happy family and social circumstances" (Rawls 1971, 74). Thus, if people exhibit a lack of motivation, it is not clear that they should be endowed with less of a share of primary goods because, in essence, it really is not their fault. Needless to say, relying on such criteria to carry out policy could result in a very large sacrifice of efficiency.

- Equalizing resources does not necessarily solve people's problems because they still might not be born with the wherewithal to use these resources in a manner than will be of benefit to them. In fact, some people might need more resources than others (e.g., the disabled).

Other Conceptions of Welfare

One reason that *A Theory of Justice* was such an important book is that it allowed others, who may not have totally agreed with Rawls, to formulate their own bases for thinking about alternative conceptions of social welfare. Rawls poked a number of holes in the utilitarian philosophy; since then others have enlarged them. A few key ideas will be presented here. Those interested in pursuing the topic may wish to consult the references for additional reading.[7]

The Role of Equality.
It is often difficult for readers to understand why philosophers might not believe that people should be granted full property rights over the resources that they have inherited and/or earned. Rawls (1971) states that "[n]o one deserves his greater natural capacity nor merits a more favorable starting place in society" (p. 102), and interestingly, most philosophers and even many economists, agree. Arrow (1983), in writing about Rawls's books, notes that under the theory,

> [e]ven natural advantages, superiorities of intelligence or strength, do not in themselves create any claims to greater rewards. . . . Personally, I share fully with this value judgment. . . . But a contradictory position—that an individual is entitled to what he creates—is widely and unreflectively held; when teaching elementary economics, I have had considerable difficulty in persuading the students that this *productivity principle* is not completely self-evident. (pp. 98–99)

The literature on moral philosophy is very clear that in creating a fair society, something must be equalized. Amartya Sen (1992) provides a reason:

> It may be useful to ask *why* it is that so many altogether different substantive theories of the ethics of social arrangements have the common feature of demanding equality of *something*—something important. It is, I believe, arguable that to have any kind of plausibility, ethical reasoning on social matters must involve elementary equal consideration for all at *some* level that is seen as critical. The absence of such equality would make a theory arbitrarily discriminating and hard to defend. A theory must accept—indeed demand—inequality in terms of many variables, but in defending those inequalities it would be hard to duck the need to relate them, ultimately, to equal consideration for all in some adequately substantial way. (p. 17)

---

7. Some especially useful books about this topic have been written by Amartya Sen (1987, 1992). Other readings are also noted.

Sen notes that even Nozick's (1974) libertarian philosophy (described above) does call for the equalization of something—libertarian rights.

Unfortunately, deciding that something ought to be equalized does not solve most of our problems. Rather, it seems to raise more questions than it answers. The main problem, of course, is that it does not tell us *what* should be equalized. Before confronting this, it is important to distinguish between two similar-sounding, but quite different concepts: "equality" and "equity." The former implies equal shares of something; the latter, a "fair" or "just" distribution, which may or may not result in equal shares.

In economics, the difference between the two terms can be seen by examining the two common forms of equity: horizontal equity and vertical equity. Horizontal equity implies that similar people are treated the same with respect to some characteristic (the choice of which is a major issue in itself)—what we are referring to here as equality. But vertical equity is much different; it is, according to Gavin Mooney (1996), "the unequal but equitable treatment of unequals" (p. 99). For example, we might, in the name of equity, establish a lower tax rate for the poor than for the rich.

The distinction among all of these terms is illustrated by Deborah Stone (1996), who discusses how to divide up and distribute "a delicious bittersweet chocolate cake" among students in her public policy class. One way, of course, is to give equal slices to all, but that seemingly fair method may lead to protests that "equality" does not result in an "equitable" distribution. Some possible objections to equal slices noted by Stone, each of which results in a different distribution of cake, include:

- Everyone in the university should get a slice, not just class members.
- Higher-ranked persons deserve bigger slices (or more frosting).
- Because males traditionally have had less access to homemade cake, each sex should get half the cake to divide among their members.
- Those who were given smaller main courses should get more cake.
- People who can't appreciate the cake should get less (or none).
- *Access* to the cake, not the cake itself, should be equalized by giving everyone a fork; competition for the cake would then ensue.
- The cake should be distributed by lottery.
- The allocation should be decided on by voting.

It is not hard to come up with close analogies to each of these arguments when allocating scarce medical goods and services.

As noted above, to be persuasive in issues involving resource allocation, it is necessary to advocate the equalization of something. What is being equalized under utilitarianism? The answer is not as straightforward as it might seem because, as noted earlier, the concept embraces several different formulations. In general, though, utilitarianism is not about equalizing something so much as maximizing something else (Sen 1992). Under classical utilitarianism, the sum of all individuals' utility is being maximized. Under ordinal utilitarianism, society is best off when each individual succeeds in maximizing his own utility, although some income redistribution is likely to be necessary to maximize the social welfare function.

We are most concerned with ordinal utilitarianism because it forms the basis of modern economics. What is being equalized under ordinal utilitarianism? One possibility is that each individual's interests are being treated equally; my utility counts as much as yours.[8] Another possibility might be that people have equal rights to produce and trade in order to maximize their utility. This is not to say that they have equal ability or opportunity to do so. Rather, in a competitive market, there are no explicit restrictions on participating in the marketplace. It is not hard to see why moral philosophers, in considering the vagaries of social advantage in the real world, would view this concept as wanting.

What, then, should be equalized? As before, no attempt will be made to review this literature; those seeking additional information should consult some of the references listed in the footnotes.[9] One line of thought, advocated by Ronald Dworkin (1981), is that people's "resources" should be equalized—a philosophy that would appear to be not terribly different from Rawls's equalization of primary goods.[10]

Another line of thought, by John Roemer (1995), is that people's "opportunity" should be equalized. The idea is that people should be responsible for their own actions once a "level playing field" is established. To operationalize this, Roemer distinguishes between factors that are beyond a person's control, and factors that are within a person's control. He gives the following example. Suppose we want to compensate people when they contract lung cancer (so that, perhaps, they can afford their medical care). We first come up with a list of factors over which people have little control; examples Roemer uses are age, ethnicity, gender,

---

8. Gavin Mooney, personal communication.

9. Two goods sources that contain a thorough set of references are Sen (1992) and Hausman and McPherson (1993).

10. Dworkin (1981) devotes several pages to explaining the difference between his theory and Rawls's theory. One difference is that Dworkin claims that his theory is tailored to the individual, whereas Rawls focuses on one representative person in a social class. It would also appear that individuals are more responsible for their actions (how they spend their resources) under Dworkin than under Rawls.

and occupation. We then look at smoking behavior within these sub-groups. Suppose that the average 60-year-old, male, black steel worker has smoked for 30 years, and the average 60-year-old, female, white college professor has smoked for 8 years. Using these figures provides a way to gauge the behaviors of others who fall into these subgroups. If we then have a black steel worker and a white professor contracting lung cancer, and they have smoked for 20 years and 15 years, respectively, the steel worker would receive more compensation—because his behavior was more responsible *given the circumstances over which he had little or no control.*

A final candidate for equalization, advocated by Sen (1992), will be particularly relevant in Section 5.3.2, under health applications. This is the equalization of capabilities, which "reflect a person's freedom to choose between alternative lives" (Sen 1992, 83). The idea here is to give people the wherewithal to be able to achieve the things they want. Capabilities focus not on resources themselves, but on what resources can do for a person.

Equalizing capabilities is different than the other systems of equalization discussed earlier. It differs from Rawls's theory, and from equalizing resources, because under those systems people are given physical resources but not necessarily the ability to use them to achieve what they want. And it differs from equality of opportunity because giving people an opportunity does not necessarily mean that they will be able to use it effectively to their own advantage. Equality of capabilities might mean that more resources would be given to a disabled person because that person could need more in order to be capable of achieving his or her goals. Or it might mean actually giving unskilled laborers the skills to achieve more—rather than simply plying them with cash grants.

Alternative Concepts of Utility

Economists do not typically inquire into why people derive utility from particular goods. Modern theory is interested simply in which bundle of goods a person prefers; the preference need not be justified. An economic system that is best able to satisfy such preferences is desirable because the preferences themselves are beyond questioning. Sen (1992) has deemed this a "welfarist" viewpoint: the only thing that matters in evaluating an economic system is how well it satisfies these preferences.

Many objections to this viewpoint can be raised; a few were mentioned in Chapter 3:

- It essentially sanctions preferences that we might view as immoral; for example, equal favor is given to those preferences that may involve harming others as compared to those that we might find to be more lofty. In this regard, Mark Sagoff (1986) writes, "It cannot be argued that the satisfaction of preferences is a good thing in itself, for many preferences are sadistic, envious, racist, or unjust (p. 302).

- It also sanctions preferences that might be, in some sense, faulty (e.g., behaviors that are self-destructive). One example is shortsightedness. Sagoff writes, "Literary and empirical studies amply confirm what every mature adult discovers: happiness and well-being come from overcoming or outgrowing many of our desires more than from satisfying them (p. 304).

- It focuses on goods rather than other values such as freedom. This leads to the seemingly faulty prediction that people will be equally happy with a particular bundle of goods that is assigned to them, versus the same bundle that they freely choose (Hahnel and Albert 1990).

It turns out that this conception of utility also does a poor job in predicting other aspects of people's behavior. One concerns why people even bother to vote. Given the infinitesimally small chance that your vote would decide an election, why go to all the effort? Another example is income taxes. Why be honest when it is so easy to cheat and so hard to be caught (Aaron 1994)? As a final illustration, it is useful to summarize Howard Margolis's (1982) discussion of people's contributions to charity.

Suppose that a public radio station embarks on a fundraising campaign, and you decide to contribute $10 (but not $11); that is, you maximize your utility by spending $10 for this charity in the place of spending it on other goods and services you could purchase. But just as you are about to call in your pledge, the station announces that someone else has just given $10. Under the conventional model, this new information will make you will forgo your contribution—the station is already $10 richer; you can now keep the $10 and be that much better off than before. Not contributing allows you to have your (bittersweet chocolate) cake and eat it too.

If people really behaved this way, then there would be no way public radio (or for that matter, almost any charity) could exist. Once a single, large donor announced his or her intention to contribute, then it would be nearly impossible to get anyone else to contribute. Everyone else would "free ride" on this donation. The outcome would be economically inefficient because far less would be contributed to charity than is desired by the public.

Fortunately, something still drives people to contribute to charities. In order to explain paradoxes such as these, it is necessary to have a broader definition of utility. An example from Chapter 2 was Sen's use of people's recycling behavior as an example of commitment—a behavior that people engage in, even though it does not seem to be in their self-interest. Another formulation is from Margolis (1982), who explains people's behavior by positing that they have two distinct altruistic motivations. One, which he calls "goods altruism," is the one we normally conceive; people receive utility when other, less well-off people have more goods to consume. The other is "participation altruism," a very different concept. Under it, people receive utility from the act of giving resources away (including their time) because it makes them feel good about themselves. This dual form of altruism, according to Margolis, can explain the paradoxes discussed earlier (why a person would vote, give to charity, not cheat on taxes).

More recently, Henry Aaron (1994) has provided a critique of utility theory, calling for "a new economics of human behavior." Although it was beyond the scope of his work to spell out the details, he believes that

> each person [has] more than one, possibly many, utility functions. In one or more of these sub-functions the arguments, as in standard theory, are particular goods and services. In others the arguments are intangible objectives such as adherence to duty, altruism, or spite, characteristics necessary for reputation or self-respect. Particular economic commodities may enter more than one function. In contrast to standard theory, however, the marginal utility of a given object may vary widely in different utility functions and may even have different signs. (pp. 15–16)

Cash versus In-Kind Transfers

One of the most common applications of ordinal utility theory is the supposed superiority of cash over in-kind transfers. The argument is as follows. Suppose that society wishes to transfer wealth from wealthier to poorer individuals, and there are two choices: giving people money or giving them goods or services directly. The former would always be superior because, by letting people choose exactly how to spend their money, they are able to maximize their utility (i.e., reach their highest affordable indifference curve). In contrast, if goods or services are provided, it would be almost impossible to maximize utility. We could never do better than through transferring cash, and could only do as well if the goods transferred were *exactly* what would have been purchased had the grant been in the form of cash.

The issue, to most economists, is one of consumer sovereignty. Should we let people make their own choices, or alternatively, should we act paternalistically by telling people how they should spend the resources that are redistributed to them? As was made clear in Chapter 3 and early in this chapter, ordinal utilitarianism has a clear preference for cash transfers because it assumes that people will make choices that are in their best interest.

One obvious issue that arises is whether people will really spend money in a way that is best for them. For example, suppose that a person is ill; society feels sympathy and gives that person $5,000. If the person takes the money and spends it on frills, alcohol, or the like, can we really say that the person is better off than having the care that the money would have purchased? Although this is certainly an important question, it will not be dealt with here, since issues like it were discussed at some length in Chapter 3. Rather, in this section we will assume that however the person spends the money will indeed maximize his or her utility.

It turns out that there are three other reasons to believe that providing goods and services may indeed be superior to providing cash; each will be addressed briefly in the following subsections.

The desires of donors. The first, and probably the most important reason, is that the superiority of cash over in-kind subsidies is based on the following propositions being true:

- we do not care about the utility of the people who make the donations (or pay the taxes); or
- we do care about the donors, but they do not care about how the money is spent.

Because these two issues are related, we will deal with them together.

Why should we ignore the wishes of the donors? One possibility is that how the recipients spend the money is none of the donors' business. But this belief contradicts a tenet of economic theory—that preferences simply exist and do not have to be justified. If donors do indeed care about how the money is being spent, then this element must be taken into account in determining what is in society's best interest. And if total welfare is simply the sum of all individuals' welfare, it is incumbent on the analyst to consider everyone's preferences, including those of the donors.

What, then, do donors care about? In considering this problem, George Daly and Fred Giertz (1972) posit that, in providing transfer payments to those who are less well off, there are two kinds of (positive consumptive) externalities to be considered. One, which they call a "goods externality," exists when the donor obtains utility from a recipient having specific goods such as housing, food, education, or health services. The other, labeled a "utility externality," is when the donor cares only about the recipient's utility, not the goods via which this utility is obtained.

The question that Daly and Giertz pose is this: "Do people, individually or collectively, extend aid to others in hopes of improving the real welfare of the recipients or in order to alter their consumption pattern?" (p. 135). To answer it, they observe people's preferences in private charity, where donations are purely voluntary, and they find that private charities "almost invariably redistribute it in the form of particular commodities" (p. 135). Furthermore, when one looks at the support for public redistribution programs (e.g., housing support), the justification is often explicitly to alter recipients' consumption patterns. In this regard, the authors add,

> [A] majority of voters might approve of public housing for slum areas but be strongly opposed to the transfer of money to people living in those slums. . . . For donors the crucial issue may be not the level of well being achieved by the recipient but rather *how* he achieves it. (p. 146)

Although some people may claim that they are only interested in the utility of the recipient, such an attitude seems a bit farfetched, as suggested in the following quotation by David Collard (1978):

> The overwhelming weight of impressionistic evidence is that people are concerned less with other people's incomes or utilities than with their consumption of specific commodities. Any reader who believes himself to be entirely non-paternalistic in his concern is asked to perform the following mental experiment. I notice that my neighbour is badly fed and badly clothed so I give him some money which he then spends on beer and tobacco. Do I feel entirely happy about this or do I somehow feel that my intentions have been thwarted? (p. 122)

Ensuring sufficient donations.   As was shown in Section 2.2.2, when there are positive externalities of consumption, then it is necessary to transfer income to ensure an economically efficient, Pareto-optimal outcome. But now suppose that donors, fearing that recipients will squander their donations, decide not to give (or vote to reduce taxes). This reduces donations to a level that is less than economically efficient. By allowing for in-kind rather than cash subsidies (and very illiquid ones at that!), more money is likely to be donated, resulting in a more efficient outcome (Daly and Giertz 1972).

Improving productivity.   Another topic raised in Chapter 2 was the fact that there are few, if any, "neutral" transfer payments. In general, taxes and subsidies result in a work disincentive that will result in a less-than-optimal amount of production. Readers are well aware of the fact that welfare payments may reduce the incentive to work because, as earned income rises, welfare payments decline.

A. C. Pigou (1932), in his classic book, *The Economics of Welfare*, raises an important reason why in-kind transfers might be superior to cash:

[T]ransference of objects not capable of being sold or pawned, and designed to satisfy needs, which, apart from the transference, a recipient would have left unsatisfied, have a different effect. The last unit of money which a man earns for himself in industry will be required to satisfy the same needs, and will, therefore, be desired with the same intensity as it would have been if no transference had been made. Hence no contraction will occur in the contribution which, by work and waiting, he makes to the national dividend. (pp. 725–726)

This point has apparently been overlooked by most analysts: if we provide a good or service to a person that would not have been purchased otherwise, then there is no work disincentive. (An example would be medical care services that a poor person could not otherwise have afforded.) Some important health applications arising from the issues raised in this section are dealt with next.

5.3 Implications for Health Policy

This chapter has focused on problems with the concept of ordinal utilitarianism, the key tool in the economics of social welfare. By relying on it, the field has been able to sidestep issues of great importance to societies, such as determining what is a fair and equitable allocation of resources. In addition, the concept was shown to be flawed because of its inability to predict such basic things as reasons why people contribute to charitable causes, and the nature of these contributions. Based on the above critique, this section provides three implications for redistributive policy in the health area.

5.3.1 Providing Health Services Rather than Cash

The last part of Section 5.2.2 showed several reasons to believe that it is better to implement redistributive policies by providing services rather than cash. This is, of course, in sharp contrast to the predictions of the conventional economic model, which posits that cash contributions will always be superior.

Needless to say, most health policymakers have eschewed the model. What they have tended to do, instead, is provide insurance coverage or reimbursement for services. No countries rely on giving low-income people money and leaving them the choice of purchasing or not purchasing health coverage.

Further evidence is provided by examining how redistribution policy is carried out in the one industrialized country that has not adopted national health insurance: the United States. In 1992, $290 billion in cash and noncash benefits was provided to persons with low income in the United States. Of this amount, only 24 percent was cash aid. The remaining 76 percent was for the direct provision of goods and services such as medical care, food, and housing. In fact, nearly twice as much was spent on providing just one in-kind service—medical care—than was spent on cash subsidies (U.S. Department of Commerce 1995).

The provision of health insurance coverage is not exactly the same as providing services directly, however. Unlike the latter, where the recipient is given no choice, when a person has health insurance he or she can choose the types of services to be received—so long as they are among the menu of services covered by the insurance program. In that respect, insurance coverage bears some resemblance to cash. But these choices are limited to a specified set of health-related goods. As discussed earlier in the chapter, donors (private charity) and taxpayers (public programs) would be unlikely to tolerate having recipients spend these resources on non-health-related items.

Thus, we see that social policy, worldwide, is conducted in a manner that is not consistent with what is predicted by the standard economic model. And, except in the United States, countries have gone the extra step of providing guaranteed health insurance coverage for the entire population, an issue considered in Section 5.3.3, national health insurance.

5.3.2 Focusing on People's Health, Not Utility

Under the conventional economic model, society strives to allow people to maximize their utility. This is because, under utilitarianism, social welfare is simply the aggregate of individual utilities. Because utility is purely subjective, not directly measurable, and not comparable across different people, public intervention is typically not advised. Rather, people should choose to spend their resources in whatever manner they think will maximize their welfare.

But as argued above, utilitarianism suffers from various shortcomings, one of which is that it is silent on a basic issue of social justice: people should not be penalized over things about which they have little or no control. It was argued that, for a theory to have any moral sway, something very important needs to be equalized. It was further argued that this "something" has to do with people's opportunities, or alternatively, their capabilities to achieve their life goals.

For decades, health economists have debated whether there is something "different" about health.[11] Much of this literature has focused on informational problems—certainly an important issue, but not terribly convincing because there are major (although perhaps not quite as severe) information problems in other sectors of the economy. Other literature has focused on the fact that there are perhaps stronger positive externalities associated with health. Arrow (1963b), for example, has stated, "The taste for improving the health of others appears to be stronger than for improving other aspects of their welfare" (p. 954). Although this provides perhaps a somewhat stronger case for health being special, one can still imagine other things—food, education, housing—that are equally compelling.

Rather, what would appear to be truly different about health concerns opportunities and capabilities: good health provides people with the opportunity and/or capability to achieve other desired things. As A. J. Culyer (1993) has written, "One reason for such beliefs may be to do with the important role [things like health] have in enabling people to fulfill their potential as persons" (p. 300). Such a viewpoint is consistent with the reason given by Lester Thurow (1977): "society's interest in the distribution of medical care springs, not from unspecified externalities that affect private-personal utility, but from our individual-societal preferences that "human rights" include *equal* "right" to health care" (p. 93).

The idea that there are other, nonutility aspects of welfare that society should consider has been coined as the "extra-welfarist" approach. (Under a welfarist approach, only individual levels of utility matter to society.) In health, these nonutility aspects have to do with either access to health services, good health itself, or both.[12] Some researchers, such as Lu Ann Aday, Ronald Andersen, and Gretchen Fleming (1980), have advocated that access to health services is the key dimension of equity, whereby "[t]he greatest 'equity' of access is said to exist when need, rather than structural or individual factors, determine[s] who gains entry to the health care system" (p. 26). More recent work by Mooney et al. (1991) appears consistent with this viewpoint. They advocate "equal access for equal need," because this "provides individuals with the *opportunity* to use needed health services" (p. 479).

Other analysts, notably Culyer (1989), have advocated that health status rather than access to care be considered the key outcome,[13] and

---

11. See, for example, Pauly (1978) as well as the following Comment by Reinhardt (1978).

12. For a good discussion of the pros and cons of equalizing health, utilization, or access, see Chapter 5 of Mooney (1994).

13. Some of Culyer's more recent writing has begun to move away from this position. In Culyer (1993), he writes: "I now think that it is more helpful in studies of distribution to focus on the

the determinants of health as the key research issue.[14] If one considers health rather than utility as an outcome, the meaning of economic efficiency is very different from the one typically used in economics. Under this conception, Culyer (1993) states that efficiency is achieved "by prioritizing the more 'urgent' and so distributing health between A and B that, at the margin, the cost of A's and B's additional health is equal to the social value attached to the health of each" (p. 312).[15]

Under this sort of allocation rule, we are interested not so much in what people demand as in how much of an improvement in health can be purchased with a given amount of money—a very nonwelfarist viewpoint. Both this view, and the one centered on access to care, seem to dictate health policy worldwide much more so than the conventional economic model. The view that centers on access as the key outcome is consistent with the fact that most government-sponsored programs seek to equalize people's ability to obtain needed medical care. The view that focuses on health itself as the key outcome forms the basis of the growing reliance on cost-effectiveness analyses in health-related studies, and on the relatively new focus on clinical outcomes and effectiveness in the field of health services research.

In contrast, what is worrisome about some of the recent developments, not only in the United States but in other countries as well, is a renewed interest in rationing the use of services by higher out-of-pocket price. (Medical savings accounts, discussed in Section 3.3.2, are one obvious example.) Such policies may indeed turn out to be effective in quelling the use of services; according to conventional theory, these policies will lead to more efficient economic outcomes if people choose to forgo services that they do not find very useful. But if one views access to health services, or health itself, as the outcome society is trying to maximize (per dollar of expenditures), then the results could be very different. By inhibiting economic access, policies aimed at reducing demand may, at the same time, lead to reductions in access, health status, or both, to levels below those that society deems optimal.

---

need for health care than on the need for health. . . . [Adam] Wagstaff and I have also come to a stipulative definition of need as 'the minimum resources required to exhaust an individual's capacity to benefit from health care'" (p. 318).

14. For a thorough model of the determinants of health, see Evans and Stoddart (1990).

15. A perhaps similar view is advocated by Alan Williams (1997), called the "fair innings" argument. He writes that this "reflects the feeling that everyone is entitled to some 'normal' span of health. . . . The implication is that anyone failing to achieve this has in some sense been cheated, whilst anyone getting more than this is 'living on borrowed time'" (p. 119). One implication is that more medical resources should be devoted to the young, who have not yet had their fair innings, with correspondingly less spent on the elderly.

5.3.3 National Health Insurance

In Section 3.3.1, it was shown that comprehensive national health insurance is not necessarily economically inefficient. Here, we consider some equity rather than efficiency issues.

If, as was just argued, societies believe that either equal access to health services or equal access to good health, is necessary in the name of social justice, then there is a clear-cut justification for national health insurance. Recent research on views about equity in several developed countries, conducted by Wagstaff et al. (1993), show that such programs are consistent with the prevailing ethical viewpoints in nearly all developed countries.[16] To reproduce their quotation (which appeared earlier, in Chapter 2), they report that

> [t]here appears to be broad agreement . . . among policy-makers in at least eight of the nine European countries [studied] that payment towards health care should be related to ability to pay rather than to use of medical facilities. Policy-makers in all nine European countries also appear to be committed to the notion that all citizens should have access to health care. In many countries this is taken further, it being made clear that access to and receipt of health care should depend on need, rather than ability to pay. (Wagstaff and van Doorslaer 1992, 363)

The one country without a national health insurance program is the United States; *why* this is the case has been debated for decades and will only be briefly touched on here. One possible reason is that there may indeed be a somewhat different ethic in the United States than in other countries. In a survey reported on by Robert Blendon and his colleagues (1995b), it was found that only 23 percent of Americans agreed with the statement, "It is the responsibility of the government to take care of the very poor people who can't take care of themselves." The numbers for other countries were considerably higher: 50 percent of Germans agreed with the statement, as did 56 percent of Poles, 62 percent of British and French, 66 percent of Italians, and 71 percent of Spaniards (Blendon et al. 1995b).

This corresponds with the findings of Wagstaff and van Doorslaer (1992) on the actual amount of equity in different countries. With regard to finance, the United States, which relies on private insurance, was the least equitable of ten countries studied; the results with regard to the equity of service delivery are less easy to generalize. Thus, there is an (albeit somewhat simplistic) argument to be made that, in eschewing universal

---

16. For a summary of research on this topic, see van Doorslaer, Wagstaff, and Rutten (eds.), 1993.

health insurance coverage, the United States is accurately reflecting an ethic of its citizenry.

Suppose that most of the U.S. public does not favor universal coverage, given its cost. This raises a most interesting question: should policymakers respect these wishes, or alternatively, still attempt to achieve universal coverage? In a discussion of these issues between Mark Pauly and Uwe Reinhardt, Pauly (1996) suggests that voters could probably be convinced that the value of certain reforms aimed at reducing the rate of uninsurance is worth the costs. However, he asserts that, "If we cannot convince the decisive voters of the value of what we value, then I think we need to accept the verdict of democracy (p. 14). Reinhardt (1996) takes a very different view. Citing a number of instances in which the policy elites prevailed over the citizenry to abolish unjust laws, he states,

> I, for one, believe that, if this nation is ever to have truly universal health insurance coverage and a truly humane safety net all around, an elite espousing those goals would have to impose that state of affairs on a generally confused plebs that has quite unstable, often logically inconsistent and utterly malleable preferences on this matter. (p. 24)[17]

National health insurance nevertheless makes a great deal of sense when one considers the alternative conceptions of social welfare that were discussed previously. If, as Margolis and Aaron argue, people have more than one element in their utility functions—if, in addition to regular "goods-based" utility, they also derive satisfaction from helping others— then they derive utility from being part of a society that helps those who do not have access to health services or good health.

In this regard, Mooney (1996) writes that

> [i]ndividuals recognise that they are members of a society and that they get some form of utility or increased well-being from being in a society, being able to make a contribution to that society, and being an active participant in that society. The source of this form of utility seems much more to be non-individualistic or at least stemming from a recognition on part of the individual that he or she is a member of a society and that such membership does convey certain benefit but also perhaps certain responsibilities. (p. 100)

This attitude has been denoted by the term, "communitarianism," where, as applied to health, there is a "desire on part of the members of that society to create a just health care service as part of a wider just

---

17. Support for this viewpoint is provided from survey data (Blendon et al. 1994), which shows that Americans' support for national health reform is quite volatile, depending in large part on the specific messages they receive from special interest advertisements.

society" (Mooney 1996, 101).[18] A key element in enacting the appropriate type of health system for a particular country is determining the extent to which the country's population holds such an ethic—a fruitful area for future research.[19]

In summary, the case for a national health insurance program that guarantees universal coverage is very strong. Universal coverage is consistent with prevailing notions of fairness; people should not be penalized for circumstances—such as their sociodemographic background or their current state of health—over which they may have little control. (The case for providing coverage to all children is especially compelling since they are *clearly* not responsible for the circumstances in which they find themselves.) In addition, unlike other characteristics, good health is instrumental in allowing people to have the capabilities to achieve their personal goals. Consequently, financial barriers to obtaining care are doubly unfair because they not only result in poorer health, but they also frustrate people's ability to attain the other things that they value. Furthermore, most people would appear to be endowed with a communitarian spirit in which they draw pride in being part of a society in which the well-being of others is an important part of their own welfare. It is thus no surprise that nearly every developed nation is committed to providing health insurance to its population, regardless of the individual's ability to pay.

---

18. A related area of inquiry is how people's sense of community affects their attitudes. In a study conducted among 1,200 Florida residents, Ahern, Hendryx, and Siddharthan (1996) found that a person's positive or negative feelings about his or her community was the best predictor of that person's perceived experiences with the health system.

19. For an extensive discussion of these issues, see Mooney (1996).

6

CONCLUSION

T HE THEME of this book has been much different from that of other health economics texts. Other texts generally accept that, unless there is strong evidence to the contrary, relying on market competition will result in the best outcomes—at least with regard to efficiency. For example, one book that the author regards highly notes:

> The use of our economic tools may lead to predictions that turn out to be different than what we observe. . . . When predictions differ from what we observe . . . , it does not mean that the theory is wrong or not useful. Instead, it is an indication that one or more of the assumptions underlying the theory have been violated. . . . When the underlying assumptions are different from what is expected, there is a possible role for public policy. (Feldstein 1988, pp. 593–94)

This statement would appear—at least to most economists—to be eminently reasonable. Since economic theory shows that market competition will lead to Pareto-optimal outcomes, why not allow market forces to operate unencumbered by government interference, unless we have solid evidence that such intervention will result in better outcomes?

This book has taken (and justified, we hope) an entirely different approach. To understand this approach, it is necessary to give close consideration to the above quotation. Feldstein indeed allows for a role for government but *only* if we observe that the predictions of economic theory differ from our observations. In particular:

- The onus is on those who would contend that market forces will not result in the best outcomes.

- In order to justify government involvement, it is necessary to demonstrate that reality differs from the predictions of the theory.

One of the main themes of this book is that the above viewpoint, which pervades economic thought, is not the right way to approach the study of health economics and the formulation of health policy. There is no reason for supposing that a competitive marketplace will result in superior outcomes in the health area, so it is not necessary to have to demonstrate that market outcomes from the operation of a hypothetical competitive market will be different from what theory would predict.

Why is there no reason to believe that a competitive marketplace will result in the best outcomes? Because such a conclusion is based on many strong assumptions being met. In this book, we have examined over a dozen of the assumptions that need to be fulfilled to ensure that a free market results in the best outcomes for society; we found that none of them is even close to being met in health. But if these assumptions are not met, economic theory provides no basis for assuming the superiority of competitive approaches. Thus, the burden of proof should not fall on those who profess the superiority of alternative approaches.

To clarify this point, suppose a country is confronting a very important health policy decision: whether to enact limits on how much it will spend each year on health-related goods and services. The above quotation implies that such a policy should be considered only if costs under a truly competitive marketplace are higher than would be predicted by theory. But even if true, this would be very difficult to demonstrate because it involves trying to answer a "counterfactual"[1] question: How much would a perfectly competitive market spend on health services? Because an answer to this question is hardly obvious and would be the subject of much dispute, the above mind-set makes it nearly impossible to justify most government involvement in health.

A better approach to policymaking does not put the burden of proof on those believing that government intervention is justified. Rather, all alternative policies being considered would start on an equal basis. Then, empirical evidence would be gathered to determine the likely effect of each alternative being considered. In the global budget example, one would need to predict the effect of enacting (versus not enacting) such a policy on costs, quality and outcomes, people's waiting time, and so on, and then weigh these various effects together to determine which policy is likely to be superior. It is possible that such an analysis would find that global budgets are not a good idea—but such a conclusion would

---

1. See Section 3.2.2 for a further discussion of counterfactual questions.

be reached after, not before, conducting the research. Competitive (i.e., noninterventionist) approaches would not be *presumed* superior.

This distinction in approach may seem niggling to some, but it turns out to be fundamental. Viewing competition as just one possible policy alternative, instead of the presumed superior policy, opens up any number of possible policies that could indeed show themselves to be superior. Many such examples were given throughout the book; they are discussed in Section 4.3, which provides a number of possible supply-side interventions.

In the conventional model, there are actually very few levers available to policymakers who are interested in health services. Because such a model is driven by consumer demand, the primary tools involve influencing demand, either by changing out-of-pocket price, or by providing additional information to consumers. There is no place to influence supply because the model presumes that suppliers will simply produce those things that are demanded.

What we see in health policy throughout the world, however, is the reliance instead on supply-side policies. These include such policy tools as capitation, DRGs, utilization review, practice guidelines, technology controls, and global budgets—just to name a few. None of these policies arises from the competitive model, nor would any be shown by economic theory to result in superior outcomes. Nevertheless, many people would argue that these supply-side policies have resulted in superior outcomes in the health services marketplace.

Determining which policies are indeed superior, however that may be defined, is a challenging task. The answers, of course, will vary depending on the particular circumstances (e.g., the disease, the population group, the country). Health services and health policy researchers throughout the world are key participants in this undertaking, and provide critically important information. But in order to prescribe the best possible set of policy options, these researchers must employ tools that expand rather than narrow this set of options.

The challenges facing health policymakers—to assure that costs are kept manageable and quality remains acceptable in a world of limited budgets but expanding technological capabilities—are daunting. New and innovative ideas are essential. If analysts misinterpret economic theory as applied to health—by assuming that market forces are necessarily superior to alternative policies—then they will blind themselves to policy options that might actually be better at enhancing social welfare.

REFERENCES

Aaron, H. J. 1994. "Public Policy, Values, and Consciousness." *Journal of Economic Perspectives* 8 (2): 3–21.

Abel-Smith, B. 1992. "Cost Containment and New Priorities in the European Community." *Milbank Quarterly* 70 (3): 393–422.

Aday, L., R. Andersen, and G. V. Fleming. 1980. *Health Care in the U.S.: Equitable to Whom?* Beverly Hills, CA: Sage Publications.

Ahern, M. M., M. S. Hendryx, and K. Siddharthan. 1996. "The Importance of Sense of Community of People's Perceptions of Their Health-Care Experiences." *Medical Care* 34 (9): 911–23.

Akerlof, G. A., and W. T. Dickens. 1992. "The Economic Consequences of Cognitive Dissonance." *American Economic Review* 72 (3): 307–19.

American Hospital Association. 1994. *Hospital Statistics, 1994–95 edition*. Chicago: American Hospital Association.

Aronson, E. 1972. *The Social Animal.* San Francisco: W. H. Freeman & Co.

Arrow, K. J. 1963a. *Social Choice and Individual Values*. New York: John Wiley.

———. 1963b. "Uncertainty and the Welfare Economics of Medical Care." *American Economic Review* 53 (5): 940–73.

———. 1983. "Some Ordinalist-Utilitarian Notes of Rawls's Theory of Justice." In *Social Choice and Justice: Collected Papers of Kenneth J. Arrow*, 96–117. Cambridge, MA: Belknap Press of Harvard University Press.

Barer, M. L., R. G. Evans, and R. J. Labelle. 1988. "Fee Controls as Cost Controls: Tales from the Frozen North." *Milbank Quarterly* 66 (1): 1–64.

Bator, F. M. 1958. "The Anatomy of Market Failure." *Quarterly Journal of Economics* 52 (3): 351–79.

Becker, G. S. 1979. "Economic Analysis and Human Behavior." In *Sociological Economics*, edited by L. Levy-Garboua. Beverly Hills, CA: Sage Publications.

Becker, G. S., and K. M. Murphy. 1988. "A Theory of Rational Addiction." *Journal of Political Economy* 96 (4): 675–700.

Bentham, J. 1791. *Principles of Morals and Legislation.* London: Doubleday.

———. 1968. "An Introduction to the Principles of Morals and Legislation." In *Utility Theory: A Book of Readings,* edited by A. N. Page, 3–29. New York: John Wiley.

Berk, M. L., and A. C. Monheit. 1992. "The Concentration of Health Expenditures: An Update." *Health Affairs* 11 (4): 145–49.

Blackorby, C., and D. Donaldson. 1990. "A Review Article: The Case Against the Use of the Sum of Compensating Variations in Cost-Benefit Analysis." *Canadian Journal of Economics* 23 (3): 471–94.

Blendon, R. J., and K. Donelan. 1990. "The Public and Emerging Debate over National Health Insurance." *New England Journal of Medicine* 323 (3): 208–12.

Blendon, R. J., et al. 1990. "Satisfaction in Health Systems in Ten Nations." *Health Affairs* 9 (2): 185–92.

Blendon, R. J., et al. 1994. "The Beliefs and Values Shaping Today's Health Reform Debate." *Health Affairs* 13 (1): 274–84.

Blendon, R. J., et al. 1995a. "The Public and the Welfare Reform Debate." *Archives of Pediatric and Adolescent Medicine* 149: 1065–69.

Blendon, R. J., et al. 1995b. "Who Has the Best Health Care System? A Second Look." *Health Affairs* 14 (4): 220–30.

Boulding, K. E. 1969. "Economics as a Moral Science." *American Economic Review* 59 (1): 1–12.

Braveman, P. A., et al. 1991. "Differences in Hospital Resource Allocation among Sick Newborns According to Insurance Coverage." *Journal of the American Medical Association* 266 (23): 3300–08.

Brook, R. H., et al. 1983. "Does Free Care Improve Adults' Health?" *The New England Journal of Medicine* 309 (23): 1426–34.

Buchanan, J. M. 1977. "Political Equality and Private Property: The Distributional Paradox." In *Markets and Morals,* edited by G. Dworkin, G. Bermant, and P. G. Brow. Washington, DC: Hemisphere Publishing Corp.

Buchmueller, T. C., and P. J. Feldstein. 1996. "Consumers' Sensitivity to Health Plan Premiums: Evidence from a Natural Experiment in California." *Health Affairs* 15 (1): 143–51.

Bunker, J., and B. Brown. 1974. "The Physician-Patient as an Informed Consumer of Surgical Services." *The New England Journal of Medicine* 290 (19): 1051–55.

Burner, S. T., and D. R. Waldo. 1995. "National Health Expenditure Projections, 1994–2005." *Health Care Financing Review* 16 (1): 221–42.

Cantril, H. 1965. *The Pattern of Human Concerns.* New Brunswick, NJ: Rutgers University Press.

Chaulk, C. P. 1994. "Preventive Health Care in Six Countries: Models for Reform?" *Health Care Financing Review* 15 (4): 7–19.

Christianson, J., et al. 1995. "Managed Care in the Twin Cities: What Can We Learn?" *Health Affairs* 14 (2): 114–30.

Clement, D. G. 1994. "Access and Outcomes of Elderly Patients Enrolled in Managed Care." *Journal of the American Medical Association* 271 (19): 1487–92.

Collard, D. 1978. *Altruism and Economy: A Study in Non-Selfish Economics.* Oxford: Martin Robertson & Co.

Congressional Budget Office. 1994. *Effects of Managed Care: An Update.* Washington, DC: Congressional Budget Office.

Coulam, R. F., and G. L. Gaumer. 1991. "Medicare's Prospective Payment System: A Critical Appraisal." *Health Care Financing Review* 13 (Annual Supplement): 45–77.

Cromwell, J., and J. Mitchell. 1986. "Physician-Induced Demand for Surgery." *Journal of Health Economics* 5 (3): 293–313.

Culyer, A. J. 1982. "The Quest for Efficiency in the Public Sector: Economists Versus Dr. Pangloss." In *Public Finance and the Quest for Efficiency, Proceedings of the 38th Congress of the International Institute of Public Finance,* 39–48. Copenhagen.

———. 1989. "The Normative Economics of Health Care Finance and Provision." *Oxford Review of Economic Policy* 5 (1): 34–58.

———. 1993. "Health, Health Expenditures, and Equity." In *Equity in the Finance and Delivery of Health Care: An International Perspective,* edited by E. van Doorslaer, A. Wagstaff, and F. Rutten, 299–319. Oxford: Oxford Medical Publications.

Culyer, A. J., and A. Wagstaff. 1993. "Equity and Equality in Health and Health Care." *Journal of Health Economics* 12 (4): 431–57.

Daly, G., and F. Giertz. 1972. "Welfare Economics and Welfare Reform." *American Economic Review* 62 (1): 131–38.

Daniels, N. 1985. *Just Health Care.* Cambridge: Cambridge University Press.

Doorslaer, E. van, and A. Wagstaff. 1992. "Equity in the Delivery of Health Care: Some International Comparisons." *Journal of Health Economics* 11 (4): 389–411.

Doorslaer, E. van, A. Wagstaff, and F. Rutten (eds.). 1993. *Equity in the Finance and Delivery of Health Care: An International Perspective.* Oxford: Oxford Medical Publications.

Dranove, D. 1995. "A Problem with Consumer Surplus Measures of the Cost of Practice Variations." *Journal of Health Economics* 14 (2): 243–51.

Duan, N., et al. 1984. "Choosing Between the Sample-Selection Model and the Multi-Part Model." *Journal of Business and Economic Statistics* 2 (3): 283–89.

Duesenberry, J. S. 1952. *Income, Saving and the Theory of Consumer Behavior.* Cambridge, MA: Harvard University Press.

Dworkin, R. 1981. "What is Equality? Part 2: Equality of Resources." *Philosophy & Public Affairs* 10 (4): 283–345.

Easterlin, R. 1974. "Does Economic Growth Improve the Human Lot? Some Empirical Evidence." In *Nations and Households in Economic Growth: Essays in Honor of Moses Abramovitz,* edited by P. A. David and M. W. Reder, 89–125. New York: Academic Press.

Ellis, R. P., and T. G. McGuire. 1993. "Supply-Side and Demand-Side Cost Sharing in Health Care." *Journal of Economic Perspectives* 7 (4): 135–51.

Elster, J. 1992. *Local Justice: How Institutions Allocate Scarce Goods and Necessary Burdens*. New York: Russell Sage Foundation.

Employee Benefit Research Institute (EBRI). 1996. *Sources of Health Insurance and Characteristics of the Uninsured*. Brief No. 179. November. Washington, DC: EBRI.

Enthoven, A. 1978. "Consumer Choice Health Plan." *The New England Journal of Medicine* 298 (12): 650–58.

———. 1978. "Consumer Choice Health Plan." *The New England Journal of Medicine* 298 (13): 709–20.

———. 1980. *Health Plan: The Only Practical Solution to the Soaring Cost of Medical Care*. Reading, MA: Addison-Wesley.

———. 1988. *Theory and Practice of Managed Competition in Health Care Finance*. Amsterdam, The Netherlands: North-Holland.

Enthoven, A., and R. Kronick. 1989. "A Consumer-Choice Health Plan for the 1990s." *The New England Journal of Medicine* 320 (1): 29–37.

———. 1989. "A Consumer-Choice Health Plan for the 1990s." *The New England Journal of Medicine* 320 (2): 94–101.

Escarce, J. J. 1992. "Explaining the Association Between Surgeon Supply and Utilization." *Inquiry* 29 (4): 403–15.

———. 1993a. "Effects of Lower Surgical Fees on the Use of Physician Services under Medicare." *Journal of the American Medical Association* 269 (19): 2513–18.

———. 1993b. "Medicare Patients' Use of Overpriced Procedures Before and After the Omnibus Budget Reconciliation Act of 1987." *American Journal of Public Health* 83 (3): 349–55.

Evans, R. G. 1984. *Strained Mercy*. Toronto, Ontario: Butterworth.

———. 1983. "Health Care in Canada: Patterns of Funding and Regulation." *Journal of Health Politics, Policy and Law* 8 (1): 1–43.

———. 1986. "Finding the Levers, Finding the Courage: Lessons from Cost Containment in North America." *Journal of Health Politics, Policy and Law* 11 (4): 585–615.

———. 1990. "Tension, Compression, and Shear: Directions, Stresses, and Outcomes of Health Care Cost Control." *Journal of Health Politics, Policy and Law* 15 (1): 101–28.

Evans, R. G., E. M. A. Parish, and F. Sully. 1973. "Medical Productivity, Scale Effects, and Demand Generation." *Canadian Journal of Economics* 6 (3): 376–93.

Evans, R. G., et al. 1983. *It's Not the Money, It's the Principle: Why User Changes for Some Services and Not Others?* Vancouver: Centre for Health Services and Policy Research, University of British Columbia.

Evans, R. G., and G. L. Stoddart. 1990. "Producing Health, Consuming Health Care." *Social Science and Medicine* 31 (12): 1347–63.

Evans, R. G., M. L. Barer, and G. L. Stoddart. 1993. "The Truth about User Fees." In *Policy Option*. Montreal, Quebec: Institute for Research on Public Policy.

Fahs, M. C. 1992. "Physician Response to the United Mine Workers' Cost-Sharing Program: The Other Side of the Coin." *Health Services Research* 27 (1): 25–45.

Feldman, R., and B. Dowd. 1991. "A New Estimate of the Welfare Loss of Excess Health Insurance." *American Economic Review* 81 (1): 297–301.

———. 1993. "What Does the Demand Curve for Medical Care Measure?" *Journal of Health Economics* 12 (2): 192–200.

Feldman, R., and M. A. Morrisey. 1990. "Health Economics: A Report on the Field." *Journal of Health Politics, Policy and Law* 15 (3): 627–46.

Feldman, R., and F. Sloan. 1988. "Competition Among Physicians, Revisited." *Journal of Health Politics, Policy and Law* 13 (2): 239–61.

Feldstein, M. S. 1973. "The Welfare Loss of Excess Health Insurance." *Journal of Political Economy* 81 (2): 251–80.

Feldstein, P. J. 1988. *Health Care Economics*. New York: John Wiley.

Fielding, J. E., and P. J. Lancry. 1993. "Lessons from France—'Viva la Difference'." *Journal of the American Medical Association* 270 (6): 748–56.

Fielding, J. E., and T. Rice. 1993 "Can Managed Care Competition Solve the Problems of Market Failure?" *Health Affairs* 12 (Supplement): 216–28.

Finkler, S. A. 1979. "Cost-Effectiveness of Regionalization: The Heart Surgery Example." *Inquiry* 16 (3): 264–70.

Fishlow, A. 1965. *American Railroads and the Transformation of the Antebellum Economy*. Cambridge, MA: Harvard University Press.

Fogel, R. A. 1964. *Railroads and American Economic Growth: Essays in Econometric History*. Baltimore, MD: Johns Hopkins Press.

Fox, D. M., and H. M. Leichter. 1993. "The Ups and Downs of Oregon's Rationing Plan." *Health Affairs* 12 (2): 66–70.

Frank, R. H. 1985. *Choosing the Right Pond: Human Behavior and the Quest for Status*. New York: Oxford University Press.

Friedman, M. 1962. *Price Theory*. Chicago: Aldine Press.

Fuchs, V. 1978. "The Supply of Surgeons and the Demand for Operations." *Journal of Human Resources* 12 (Supplement): 35–56.

———. 1996. "Economics, Values, and Health Care Reform." *American Economic Review* 86 (1): 1–23.

Gabel, J. R., and G. A. Jensen. 1989. "The Price of State Mandated Benefits." *Inquiry* 26 (3): 419–31.

Gabel, J. R., and T. H. Rice. 1985. "Reducing Public Expenditures for Physician Services: The Price of Paying Less." *Journal of Health Politics, Policy and Law* 9 (4): 595–609.

Gabel, J. R., et al. 1990. "Employer-Sponsored Health Insurance, 1989." *Health Affairs* 9 (3): 161–75.

Gabel, J. R., et al. 1994. "The Health Insurance Picture in 1993: Some Rare Good News." *Health Affairs* 13 (1): 327–36.

Ginsburg, P. B., and C. Hogan. 1993. "Physician Response to Fee Changes: A Contrary View." *Journal of the American Medical Association* 269 (19): 2550–52.

Gintis, H. 1970. *Neo-Classical Welfare Economics and Individual Development.* Cambridge, MA: Union for Radical Political Economists.

Gold, M. R., et al. 1994. "A National Survey of the Arrangements Managed Care Plans Make with Physicians." *The New England Journal of Medicine* 333 (25): 1678–83.

Graaff, Jan de V. 1971. *Theoretical Warfare Economics.* London: Cambridge University Press.

Green, R. M. 1976. "Health Care and Justice in Contract Theory Perspective." In *Ethics and Health Policy*, edited by R. M. Veatch and R. Branson. Cambridge, MA: Ballinger.

Greenfield, S., et al. 1992. "Variations in Resource Utilization Among Medical Specialties and Systems of Care: Results from the Medical Outcomes Study." *Journal of the American Medical Association* 267 (12): 1624–30.

Hadley, J., J. Holahan, and W. Scanlon. 1979. "Can Fee-for-Service Reimbursement Coexist with Demand Creation?" *Inquiry* 16 (3): 247–58.

Hahnel, R., and M. Albert. 1990. *Quiet Revolution in Welfare Economics.* Princeton, NJ: Princeton University Press.

Hannan, E. L., et al. 1991. "Coronary Artery Bypass Surgery: The Relationship Between In-Hospital Mortality Rate and Surgical Volume after Controlling for Clinical Risk Factors." *Medical Care* 29 (11): 1094–1107.

Hausman, D. M., and M. S. McPherson. 1993. "Taking Ethics Seriously: Economics and Contemporary Moral Philosophy." *Journal of Economic Literature* 31 (2): 671–731.

Hay, J., and M. J. Leahy. 1982. "Physician-Induced Demand: An Empirical Analysis of the Consumer Information Gap." *Journal of Health Economics* 1 (3): 231–44.

Hay, J. W., and R. J. Olsen. 1984. "Let Them Eat Cake: A Note on Comparing Alternative Models of the Demand for Medical Care." *Journal of Business and Economic Statistics* 2 (3): 279–82.

Hayek, F. A. 1945. "The Use of Knowledge by Society." *American Economic Review* 35 (4): 519–30.

Hemenway, D., and D. Fallon. 1985. "Testing for Physician-Induced Demand with Hypothetical Cases." *Medical Care* 23 (4): 344–49.

Hester, J., and I. Leveson. 1974. "The Health Insurance Study: A Critical Appraisal." *Inquiry* 11 (1): 53–60.

Hibbard, J. H., and J. J. Jewett. 1996. "What Type of Quality Information Do Consumers Want in a Health Care Report Card?" *Medical Care Research and Review* 53 (1): 28–47.

———. 1997. "Will Quality Report Cards Help Consumers?" *Health Affairs* 16 (5): 218–28.

Hibbard, J. H., S. Sofaer, and J. J. Jewett. 1996. "Condition-Specific Performance

Information: Assessing Salience, Comprehension, and Approaches for Communicating Quality." *Health Care Financing Review* 18 (1): 95–109.

Hibbard, J. H., and E. C. Weeks. 1989a. "The Dissemination of Physician Fee Information: Impact on Consumer Knowledge, Attitudes, and Behaviors." *Journal of Health & Social Policy* 1 (1): 75–87.

———. 1989b. "Does the Dissemination for Comparative Data on Physician Fees Affect Consumer Use of Services?" *Medical Care* 27 (12): 1167–74.

Hillman, A. L., M. V. Pauly, and J. J. Kerstein. 1989. "How Do Financial Incentives Affect Physicians' Clinical Decisions and the Financial Performance of Health Maintenance Organizations?" *The New England Journal of Medicine* 321 (1): 86–92.

Hillman, A. L., W. P. Welch, and M. V. Pauly. 1992. "Contractual Arrangements Between HMOs and Primary Care Physicians: Three-Tiered HMOs and Risk Pools." *Medical Care* 30 (2): 136–48.

Hoerger, T. J., and L. Z. Howard. 1995. "Search Behavior and Choice of Physician in the Market for Prenatal Care." *Medical Care* 33 (4): 332–49.

Holahan, J., and W. Scanlon. 1979. "Physician Pricing in California: Price Controls, Physician Fees, and Physician Incomes from Medicare and Medicaid." *Grants and Contracts Report, Pub. No. 03006.* Washington, DC: Health Care Financing Administration.

Hurley, J., and R. Labelle. 1995. "Relative Fees and the Utilization of Physicians' Services in Canada." *Health Economics* 4 (6): 419–38.

Hurley, J., R. Labelle, and T. Rice. 1990. "The Relationship Between Physician Fees and the Utilization of Medical Services in Ontario." *Advances in Health Economics and Health Services Research* 11: 49–78.

Institute of Medicine. 1990. *Clinical Practice Guidelines.* Washington, DC: National Academy Press.

Isaacs, S. L. 1996. "Consumers' Information Needs: Results of a National Survey." *Health Affairs* 15 (4): 31–41.

Jensen, G. A., et al. 1997. "The New Dominance of Managed Care: Insurance Trends in the 1990s." *Health Affairs* 16 (1): 125–36.

Jewett, J. J. and J. H. Hibbard. 1996. "Comprehension of Quality Indicators: Differences Among Privately Insured, Publicly Insured, and Uninsured." *Health Care Financing Review* 18 (1): 75–94.

Jones, S. B. 1991. *Where Does Marketplace Competition in Health Care Take Us? Impressions, Issues, and Unanswered Questions from the NHPF Site Visit to Minneapolis–St. Paul.* Washington, DC: National Health Policy Forum.

Jonsson, B. 1989. "What Can Americans Learn From Europeans?" *Health Care Financing Review* 11 (Supplement): 79–109.

Katz, S. J., L. F. McMahon, and W. G. Manning. 1996. "Comparing the Use of Diagnostic Tests in Canadian and U.S. Hospitals." *Medical Care* 34 (2): 117–25.

Keeler, E. B. 1987. "Effect of Cost Sharing on Physiological Health, Health Practices, and Worry." *Health Services Research* 22 (3): 279–306.

Kransik, A., et al. 1990. "Changing Remuneration Systems: Effects on Activity in General Practice." *British Medical Journal* 300 (6741): 1698–1701.

Kuttner, R. 1984. *The Economic Illusion: False Choices Between Prosperity and Social Justice.* Boston: Houghton Mifflin.

———. 1997. *Everything for Sale: The Virtue and Limits of Markets.* New York: Alfred A. Knopf.

Labelle, R., G. Stoddart, and T. Rice. 1994. "A Re-Examination of the Meaning and Importance of Supplier-Induced Demand." *Journal of Health Economics* 13 (3): 347–68.

Leape, L. 1989. "Unnecessary Surgery." *Health Services Research* 24 (3): 351–407.

Lee, A. J., and J. B. Mitchell. 1994. "Physician Reaction to Price Changes: An Episode-of-Care Analysis." *Health Care Financing Review* 16 (2): 65–83.

Leibenstein, H. 1976. *Beyond Economic Man.* Cambridge, MA: Harvard University Press.

———. 1966. "Allocative Efficiency vs. 'X-Efficiency'." *American Economic Review* 392–415.

Levit, K. R., et al. 1985. "National Health Expenditures, 1984." *Health Care Financing Review* 7 (1): 1–35.

Levit, K. R., et al. 1996a. "National Health Expenditures, 1995." *Health Care Financing Review* 18 (1): 175–241.

Levit, K. R., H. C. Lazenby, and L. Sivarajan. 1996b. "Health Care Spending in 1994: Slowest in Decades." *Health Affairs* 15 (2): 130–44.

Light, D. W. 1995. "*Homo Economicus*: Escaping the Traps of Managed Competition." *European Journal of Public Health* 5 (3): 145–54.

Lindsey, P. A., and J. P. Newhouse. 1990. "The Cost and Value of Second Surgical Opinion Programs: A Critical Review of the Literature." *Journal of Health Politics, Policy and Law* 15 (3): 543–70.

Lipsey, R. G., and K. Lancaster. 1956–1957. "The General Theory of the Second Best." *Review of Economic Studies* 24 (1): 11–32.

Little, I. M. D. 1957. *A Critique of Welfare Economics.* London: Oxford at the Clarendon Press, Oxford University Press.

Lohr, K. N., et al. 1986. "Effect of Cost Sharing on Use of Medically Effective and Less Effective Care." *Medical Care* 24 (Supplement): S31—S38.

Luft, H. S. 1973. "The Impact of Poor Health on Earnings." *Health Care Policy Discussion Paper No. 10.* Boston: Harvard Center for Community Health and Medical Care, Program on Health Care Policy, Harvard University.

———. 1978. *Poverty and Health.* Cambridge, MA: Ballinger.

———. 1981. *Health Maintenance Organizations: Dimensions of Performance.* New York: John Wiley.

Luft, H. S., J. P. Bunker, and A. C. Enthoven. 1979. "Should Operations Be Regionalized? The Empirical Relation Between Surgical Volume and Mortality." *The New England Journal of Medicine* 301 (25): 1364–69.

Manning, W., et al. 1984. "A Controlled Trial of the Effect of a Prepaid Group Practice on Use of Services." *The New England Journal of Medicine* 310 (23): 1505–10.

Manning, W. G., et al. 1987. "Health Insurance and the Demand for Medical Care: Evidence from a Randomized Experiment." *American Economic Review* 77 (3): 251–77.

Margolis, H. 1982. *Selfishness, Altruism, and Rationality*. Cambridge: Cambridge University Press.

Marmor, T. R., and A. Dunham. 1983. "Political Science and Health Services Administration." In *Political Analysis and American Medical Care: Essays*, edited by T. R. Marmor, 3–44. London: Cambridge University Press.

Marshall, A. 1920. *Principles of Economics*. London: Macmillan and Co.

McCarthy, T. R. 1985. "The Competitive Nature of the Primary Care Physician Services Market." *Journal of Health Economics* 4 (2): 93–117.

McCormack, L. A., et al. 1996. "Medicare Beneficiary Counseling Programs: What Are They and Do They Work?" *Health Care Financing Review* 18 (1): 127–40.

Mechanic, D. 1979. *Future Issues in Health Care*. New York: The Free Press, Macmillan and Co.

———. 1990. "The Role of Sociology in Health Affairs." *Health Affairs* 9 (1): 85–97.

Milgram, S. 1963. "Behavioral Study of Obedience." *Journal of Abnormal and Social Psychology* 67 (4): 371–78.

Miller, D. 1992. "Distributive Justice." *Ethics* 102 (April): 555–93.

Miller, R. H. 1996. "Competition in the Health System: Good News and Bad News." *Health Affairs* 15 (2): 107–20.

Miller, R. H., and H. S. Luft. 1994. "Managed Care Plan Performance Since 1980: A Literature Analysis." *Journal of the American Medical Association* 271 (19): 1512–19.

Mishan, E. J. 1969a. *Welfare Economics: Ten Introductory Essays*. New York: Random House.

———. 1969b. *Welfare Economics: An Assessment*. Amsterdam, The Netherlands: North-Holland.

———. 1982. *What is Political Economy All About?* Cambridge: Cambridge University Press.

Mitchell, J. B., G. Wedig, and J. Cromwell. 1989. "The Medicare Physician Fee Freeze: What Really Happened?" *Health Affairs* 8 (1): 21–33.

Mooney, G. 1994. *Key Issues in Health Economics*. New York: Harvester Wheatsheaf.

———. 1996. "A Communitarian Critique of Health (Care) Economics." Presented at the inaugural meetings of the International Health Economics Association, Vancouver, British Columbia.

———. 1996. "And Now for Vertical Equity? Some Concerns Arising from Aboriginal Health in Australia." *Health Economics* 5 (2): 99–103.

Mooney, G., et al. 1991. "Utilisation as a Measure of Equity: Weighing Heat?" *Journal of Health Economics* 10 (4): 475–80.

Moore, F. C. 1877. *Fires: Their Causes, Prevention, and Extinction*. New York: F. C. Moore.

Nath, S. K. 1969. *A Reappraisal of Welfare Economics*. London: Routledge & Kegan Paul.

National Health Policy Forum. 1995. *Consolidation in the Health Care Marketplace and Antitrust Policy*. Washington, DC: George Washington University.

Newhouse, J. P. 1974. "The Health Insurance Study: Response to Hester and Leveson." *Inquiry* 11 (3): 236–41.

———. 1978. *The Economics of Medical Care*. Reading, MA: Addison-Wesley.

———. 1993. "An Iconoclastic View of Health Cost Containment." *Health Affairs* 12 (Supplement): 152–71.

———. 1994. "Patients at Risk: Health Reform and Risk Adjustment." *Health Affairs* 13 (1): 132–46.

Newhouse, J. P., et al. 1987. "Findings of the RAND Health Insurance Experiment—a Response to Welch et al." *Medical Care* 25 (2): 157–79.

Newhouse, J. P., et al. 1993. *Free for All? Lessons from the RAND Health Insurance Experiment*. Cambridge, MA: Harvard University Press.

Ng, Y.-K. 1979. *Welfare Economics*. London: Macmillan and Co.

Nozick, R. 1974. *Anarchy, State, and Utopia*. New York: Basic Books.

Ogden, D., R. Carlson, and G. Bernstein. 1990. "The Effect of Primary Care Incentives." *Proceedings from the 1990 Group Health Institute*. Washington, DC: Group Health Association of America.

Paul-Shaheen, P., J. D. Clark, and D. Williams. 1987. "Small Area Analysis: A Review and Analysis of the North American Literature." *Journal of Health Politics, Policy and Law* 12 (4): 741–809.

Parkin, M. 1994. *Microeconomics*. Reading, MA: Addison-Wesley.

Pauly, M. V. 1968. "The Economics of Moral Hazard: Comment." *American Economic Review* 58 (4): 531–37.

———. 1978. "Is Medical Care Different?" In *Competition in the Health Care Sector: Past, Present, and Future*, edited by W. Greenberg, 19–48. Washington, DC: Bureau of Economics, Federal Trade Commission.

———. 1996. "The Fall and Rise of Health Care Reform: A Dialogue." In *Looking Back, Looking Forward: "Staying Power" in Issues in Health Care Reform*, 7–38. Washington, DC: Institute of Medicine.

Pauly, M. V., and M. A. Satterthwaite. 1981. "The Pricing of Primary Care Physicians' Services: A Test of the Role of Consumer Information." *Bell Journal of Economics* 12 (2): 488–506.

Peter, L., and R. Hull. 1969. *The Peter Principle*. New York: William Morrow.

Phelps, C. E. 1992. *Health Economics*. New York: HarperCollins.

———. 1995a. "Perspectives in Health Economics." *Health Economics* 4 (5): 335–53.

———. 1995b. "Welfare Loss from Variations: Further Considerations." *Journal of Health Economics* 14 (2): 253–60.

Phelps, C. E., and S. T. Parente. 1990. "Priority Setting in Medical Technology and Medical Practice Assessment." *Medical Care* 29 (8): 703–23.

Phelps, C. E., and C. Mooney. 1992. "Correction and Update on Priority Setting in Medical Technology Assessment in Medical Care." *Medical Care* 30 (8): 744–51.

Physician Payment Review Commission. 1993. *Annual Report to Congress*. Washington, DC.

Pigou, A. C. 1932. *The Economics of Welfare, 4th ed*. London: Macmillan and Co.

Pilote, L., et al. 1995. "Differences in the Treatment of Myocardial Infarction Between the United States and Canada: A Survey of Physicians in the GUSTO Trial." *Medical Care* 33 (6): 598–610.

Pollak, D. A., et al. 1994. "Prioritization of Mental Health Services in Oregon." *Milbank Quarterly* 72 (3): 515–50.

Pollack, R. A. 1978. "Endogenous Tastes in Demand and Welfare Analysis." *American Economic Review* 68 (2): 374–79.

Rawls, J. 1971. *A Theory of Justice*. Cambridge, MA: Belknap Press of Harvard University.

Reinhardt, U. E. 1978. "Comment on Paper by Frank A. Sloan and Roger Feldman." In *Competition in the Health Care Sector: Past, Present, and Future*, edited by W. Greenberg, 156–90. Washington, DC: Bureau of Economics, Federal Trade Commission.

———. 1985. "The Theory of Physician-Induced Demand: Reflections After a Decade." *Journal of Health Economics* 4 (2): 187–93.

———. 1989. "Economists in Health Care: Saviors, or Elephants in a Porcelain Shop?" *American Economic Review Papers and Proceedings* 79 (2): 337–42.

———. 1992. "Reflections on the Meaning of Efficiency: Can Efficiency Be Separated from Equity?" *Yale Law & Policy Review* 10: 302–15.

———. 1996. "Comment on Mark Pauly." In *Looking Back, Looking Forward: "Staying Power" in Issues in Health Care Reform*, 7–38. Washington, DC: Institute of Medicine.

Rice, T. H. 1983. "The Impact of Changing Medicare Reimbursement Rates on Physician-Induced Demand." *Medical Care* 21 (8): 803–15.

———. 1984. "Physician-Induced Demand for Medical Care: New Evidence from the Medicare Program." *Advances in Health Economics and Health Services Research* 5: 129–60.

———. 1992a. "An Alternative Framework for Evaluating Welfare Losses in the Health Care Market." *Journal of Health Economics* 11 (1): 88–92.

———. 1992b. "Containing Health Care Costs in the United States." *Medical Care Review* 49 (1): 19–65.

Rice, T., and J. Gabel. 1996. "The Internal Economics of HMOs: A Research Agenda." *Medical Care Research and Review* 53 (Supplement): S44–S64.

Rice, T., E. R. Brown, and R. Wyn. 1989. "Holes in the Jackson Hole Approach to Health Care Reform." *Journal of the American Medical Association* 270 (11): 1357–62.

Rice, T. H., and R. J. Labelle. 1989. "Do Physicians Induce Demand for Medical Services?" *Journal of Health Politics, Policy and Law* 14 (3): 587–600.

Rice, T., and K. R. Morrison. 1994. "Patient Cost Sharing for Medical Services: A

Review of the Literature and Implications for Health Care Reform." *Medical Care Review* 51 (3): 235–87.

Rice, T., and K. E. Thorpe. 1993. "Income-Related Cost Sharing in Health Insurance." *Health Affairs* 12 (1): 21–39.

Rizzo, J. A., and D. Blumenthal. 1996. "Is the Target Income Hypothesis an Economic Heresy?" *Medical Care Research and Review* 53 (3): 243–66.

Robbins, Lord (Lionel). 1984. "Economics and Political Economy." In *An Essay on the Nature and Significance of Economic Science, 3rd ed*, xi–xxxiii. London, Macmillan Press.

Robert Wood Johnson Foundation. 1994. *Annual Report: Cost Containment.* Princeton, NJ.

Robinson, J. 1962. *Economic Philosophy.* Chicago: Aldine Publishing Company.

Rodwin, M. A. 1993. *Medicine, Money, and Morals: Physicians' Conflicts of Interest.* New York: Oxford University Press.

———. 1996. "Consumer Protection and Managed Care: The Need for Organized Consumers." *Health Affairs* 15 (3): 110–21.

Roemer, J. E. 1994. *Egalitarian Perspectives.* Cambridge, MA: Cambridge University Press.

———. 1995. "Equality and Responsibility." *Boston Review* 20 (2): 3–7.

Roemer, M. I. 1991. *National Health Systems of the World: Volume One, The Countries.* New York: Oxford University Press.

Roos, L. L., et al. 1990. "Postsurgical Mortality in Manitoba and New England." *Journal of the American Medical Association* 263 (18): 2453–58.

Roos, L. L., et al. 1992. "Health and Surgical Outcomes in Canada and the United States." *Health Affairs* 11 (2): 56–72.

Ross, L. D. 1988. "Situational Perspectives on the Obedience Experiments." *Contemporary Psychology* 33 (2): 101–104.

Ross, L., and R. E. Nisbett. 1991. *The Person and the Situation: Perspectives of Social Psychology.* Philadelphia, PA: Temple University Press.

Rowley, C. K., and A. T. Peacock. 1975. *Welfare Economics: A Liberal Restatement.* New York: John Wiley.

Rubin, H. R., et al. 1993. "Patients' Ratings of Outpatient Visits in Different Practice Settings: Results from the Medical Outcomes Study." *Journal of the American Medical Association* 270 (7): 835–40.

Rublee, D. A. 1994. "Medical Technology in Canada, Germany, and the United States: An Update." *Health Affairs* 13 (4): 113–17.

Safran, D. G., A. R. Tarlov, and W. H. Rogers. 1994. "Primary Care Performance in Fee-for-Service and Prepaid Health Care Systems: Results from the Medical Outcomes Study." *Journal of the American Medical Association* 271 (20): 1579–86.

Sagoff, M. 1986. "Values and Preferences." *Ethics* 96 (January): 301–16.

Samuelson, P. A. 1938. "A Note on the Pure Theory of Consumer Behavior." *Economica* 5 (17): 61–71.

———. 1947. *Foundations of Economic Analysis.* New York: Atheneum.

Index